THE ESSENTIAL VITAMIN K FOODS LISTS FOR WARFARIN USERS

WITH MORE THAN 1500 FOODS LISTED WITH VITAMIN K CONTENT — DETAILED MEAL PLANNING GUIDELINES

DR. H. MAHER

CONTENTS

INTRODUCTION

Warfarin (Coumadin, Jantoven) remains the mainstay for preventing arterial and venous thrombosis and the primary and secondary prevention of stroke related to atrial fibrillation. Warfarin is in the anticoagulant class of medication and decreases blood's ability to clot. This helps prevents new clots from forming and stops existing clots from growing larger. However, Warfarin's effectiveness is affected by your daily vitamin K intake. Therefore you should be consistent in how much vitamin K you get daily and aim for stable daily vitamin K intakes.

Warfarin (brand names Coumadin and Jantoven) is an anticoagulant (blood thinner) medication. It has been available in the united states since its first approval by the Food and Drug Administration (FDA) in 1954.

Warfarin is used as a valuable medication in the prophylaxis and treatment of deep vein thrombosis (DVT), pulmonary embolism (PE), atrial fibrillation (AF), and myocardial infarction.

MECHANISM OF ACTION

Warfarin is a Vitamin K antagonist—VKA that blocks vitamin K from producing some active coagulation factors in the liver, reducing the number of clotting factors in your blood and prolonging the clotting time. Warfarin lowers your blood's ability to clot but does not prevent it from clotting completely. Your blood will be less likely to form unwanted clots. If you have a blood clot, Warfarin prevents the clot from growing larger and keeps it from breaking off and moving to your brain, heart, or lung.

WHAT DOES WARFARIN TREAT?

Warfarin is commonly prescribed to:

- Prevent and manage venous thromboembolism (blood clots in the veins) and its related medical conditions, deep vein thrombosis (DVT), and pulmonary embolisms (PE).
- Prevent and treat thromboembolism in patients suffering from atrial fibrillation.
- Prevent and treat thromboembolic complications in patients who undergo mechanical heart valve replacement.
- Reduce the risk of recurrent myocardial infarction, stroke, systemic embolization after myocardial infarction

It's also prescribed to people with certain health conditions or risks to prevent blood clots from forming in their blood vessels.

USE OF INR FOR MONITORING WARFARIN TREATMENT

PT/INR stands for prothrombin time / international normalized ratio and is a type of calculation based on the results of prothrombin time (PT).

Prothrombin is a vitamin K–dependent plasma protein made by the liver. It is also referred to as factor II, one of about 13 active clotting factors in the blood. Clotting factors work together to help stop bleeding after an injury or cut. The test measures how much time it takes for a clot to form in your blood sample and will determine if Warfarin is working the way it should:

- PT/INR stays within your therapeutic range: your risk of getting a blood clot or bleeding is small.
- PT/INR is below your therapeutic range: your blood is clotting too quickly, putting you at risk for harmful blood clots.
- PT/INR is above your therapeutic range: your blood is clotting too slowly, putting you at risk of bleeding.

The PT/INR measurement is the key component in keeping good control of warfarin treatment. The target INR range is between 2 and 3. an INR below or above the range can be dangerous for the patient. The dose of warfarin should be adjusted accordingly to bring the target INR back to 2 to 3.

WHY DO YOU HAVE TO KEEP YOUR VITAMIN K LEVEL CONSISTENT?

For most patients on Warfarin therapy, vitamin K may change how Warfarin works and cause your prothrombin time (PT) test (or INR test) to change. If you eat more vitamin K, your INR will decrease, and warfarin effectiveness will be altered, putting you at risk of dangerous blood clots. If you eat less vitamin K, your INR will increase, putting you at risk of bleeding. **You don't need to stop eating foods and drinks containing vitamin K.** However, you should make informed and smarter food choices by focusing on the vitamin k content of foods and beverages. You have to avoid or restrict foods that are high in vitamin k, prefer low vitamin-k-containing foods and try to **keep the amounts from food and supplements about the same every day**.

For this reason, it's essential to be aware of the vitamin K content in all the foods you prefer and know how much you can safely eat while keeping your INR in the therapeutic range.

HOW MUCH VITAMIN K DO YOU NEED?

The daily amount of vitamin K you need depends on your age and sex. Recommended Dietary Allowances (RDAs) for vitamin k are listed below in micrograms (mcg).

- for 19+ years old males, the RDA is 120 mcg daily
- for 19+ years old females, the RDA is 90 mcg daily
- for 19+ years old pregnant female, the RDA is 90 mcg daily
- for 19+ years old lactating female, the RDA is 90 mcg daily

HOW THIS BOOK IS ORGANIZED?

"The Essential Vitamin K Foods Lists for Warfarin Users" is your indispensable guide to monitoring your Vitamin K intake and keeping your INR within its therapeutic range while taking Warfarin.

Foods are sorted alphabetically within a food category, such as "Vegetables" or "Fruit." This makes it simple to compare the sorts of foods you eat every day and helps you identify which high-Vitamin-K foods you must replace with low-Vitamin-K ones. The food categories used are:

1. Vegetables and Vegetable Products
2. Fruit and Fruit Products
3. Meats
4. Bread & Bakery Products
5. Beans and lentils
6. Finfish and Shellfish Products

PART I
THE WARFARIN THERAPY: BASICS

UNDERSTANDING BLOOD CLOTS

BLOOD CLOTTING

Blood clotting, or coagulation, is a critical process by which the body reduces and stops bleeding when you get injured. It occurs each time a blood vessel ruptures and blood starts to flow out. It involves two interrelated stages:

1. primary hemostasis, which consists of the formation of a weak plug
2. secondary hemostasis, which consists of stabilizing the formed weak plug into a blood clot

Primary Hemostasis

Primary hemostasis leads to the initial sealing of the vascular damage by forming a weak plug. It involves four sequences:

1. blood vessel constriction. Vasospasm of the damaged blood vessel is triggered by the injury and induces, in turn, the constriction of the blood vessel by small muscles in its wall,

which decreases blood flow and results in less blood leaking out.

2. platelet adhesion. When a blood vessel is damaged, collagen becomes exposed and attracts platelets—the smallest cell fragments of blood—to the injury site. Platelet adhesion is the mechanism by which platelets bind to nonplatelet surfaces.

3. platelet activation is a key process of hemostasis following adhesion. It activates platelet by agonists such as adenosine diphosphate and collagen fibers present at the sites of injury of the blood vessel. During this sequence, the shapes of platelets change from plate-like forms to extend long filaments.

4. platelet aggregation. In this final sequence. Activated platelets aggregate with each other at the site of vascular injury.

SECOND HEMOSTASIS

Secondary hemostasis refers to the sequence of enzymatic reactions that stabilize the weak platelet plug. It converts fibrinogen, a soluble protein found in the blood plasma, into an insoluble protein known as fibrin. Fibrin molecules then merge to form extended fibrin networks that enmesh platelets, building up a sponging patch that progressively solidifies and contracts to form the blood clot.

BLOOD CLOTTING DISORDER

Your bodies usually break down the formed clot after you have healed. However, clots sometimes form in veins or arteries without reason or don't dissolve after vascular damage. Thrombosis refers to the formation of a blood clot—thrombus—within a blood vessel.

Thrombosis is divided into two main types:

- arterial thrombosis occurs when one or more thrombus form, travel in the circulatory system, and **blocks an artery**—a vessel that carries blood away from your heart. Arterial blood clots can block blood flow to critical organs like the heart, lung, or brain, resulting in deadly conditions such as heart attack or stroke.
- venous thromboembolism (VTE, or venous thrombosis,) occurs when one or more blood clots form and **block a vein**— a vessel that carries blood to your heart. VTE is a medical condition that includes deep vein thrombosis (DVT) and pulmonary embolism (PE). DVT generally occurs in the leg but can also affect other parts of your body. PE happens when a clot travels through the bloodstream to the lungs artery causing blood flow blockage. This blood vessel blockage can be extremely dangerous if the clot is large.

SYMPTOMS OF BLOOD CLOTTING DISORDER

Blood clotting disorders can be life-threatening depending on which part of your body is affected by the blood clot. A blood clot generally does not have any signs until it blocks the blood flow to parts of the body.

If the blood clot blocks the coronary arteries (i.e., a heart attack occurs), the symptoms are:

- chest pain or discomfort
- jaw, neck, or back pain or discomfort
- Shortness of breath
- lightheadedness
- arms pain or discomfort
- shoulders Pain or discomfort
- tiredness

- nausea or vomiting
- shortness of breath
- dizziness

If this blood clot blocks an artery in the brain (i.e., stroke occurs), the symptoms are:

- Sudden and abrupt numbness on one side of the body
- Sudden and abrupt weakness on one side of the body
- Sudden confusion
- Abrupt trouble speaking,
- difficulty understanding speech.
- weakness in the face, arm, or leg
- Sudden trouble of vision in one or both eyes.
- confusion (stroke)
- Sudden loss of balance
- lack of coordination.

If this blood clot blocks an artery in the lung (i.e., pulmonary embolism occurs), the symptoms are:

- chest pain
- difficulty breathing,
- coughing,
- coughing up blood, and irregular heartbeats.
- shortness of breath
- sharp and abrupt chest pains
- rapid or irregular heartbeats
- unexplained cough
- hemoptysis—coughing up blood
- apprehension or anxiety
- sweating
- feeling faint
- tiredness

If this blood clot blocks a vein a the leg (i.e., Deep Vein Thrombosis occurs), the symptoms are:

- leg warm to touch
- swelling
- pain in the leg
- tenderness in the leg
- redness of the skin

HOW ARE BLOOD CLOTTING DISORDERS TREATED?

Once a patient is diagnosed with a blood clot, blood thinners, or anti-coagulants, are prescribed to reduce the blood's ability to clot. Depending on the type and location of the blood clot, the patient will often be prescribed an anticoagulant for approximately three to six months, but sometimes he will need to take the treatment for the rest of his life.

THE ANTICOAGULANT THERAPY

Vitamin K antagonists—VKAs are the most commonly prescribed anticoagulants and have a favorable benefit-risk ratio. Regular blood tests to measure the INR allow your provider to assess the effectiveness of the treatment and the absence of over or under dosage.

Anticoagulants are drugs that prevent blood clots by increasing the time it takes for blood to clot. They are prescribed to people at high risk of blood clots to lower their risk of severe conditions such as strokes, heart attacks, and pulmonary embolism. There are four main classes of anticoagulants medications:

- **Vitamin K antagonist (VKA)** works by reducing the availability of vitamin K and, consequently, the blood's ability to clot. Warfarin belongs to the VKA class and is the most widely prescribed anticoagulant in the world.
- **Factor Xa inhibitors** bind to activated factor X (Xa) to

decrease their activity, which leads to less thrombin and, consequently, less clotting.

- **Heparin** is an injectable anticoagulant that inhibits thrombin and factor Xa by activating antithrombin III.
- **Direct Thrombin inhibitor**s bind to and inhibit the activity of clotting protein thrombin which prevents blood clot formation.
- **Platelet inhibitors** inhibit platelet function, which helps reduce the formation of clots. Several classes of platelet inhibitor drugs are available such as Aspirin and Clopidogrel.

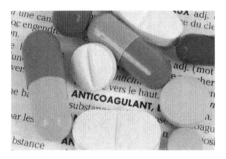

SIDE EFFECTS OF ANTICOAGULANTS

The most common side effect risk with anticoagulant therapy is excessive bleeding. Common side effects include:

- severe bruising
- prolonged nosebleeds
- bleeding gums
- heavy periods in women

Severe side effects include:

- blood in the urine
- blood in stools
- coughing up or vomiting blood

THE WARFARIN THERAPY

Warfarin therapy continues to be essential in preventing arterial and venous thrombosis and the primary and secondary prevention of stroke related to atrial fibrillation. Warfarin therapy requires carefully monitoring to avoid excessive bleeding and to ensure Warfarin is working as intended. Periodic blood testing is required to measure the patient's prothrombin time (PT) and the international normalized ratio (INR).

Warfarin (Coumadin and Jantoven) is an anticoagulant (blood thinner) medication. It has been available in the united states since its first approval by the Food and Drug Administration (FDA) in 1954.

Warfarin is used as a valuable medication in the prophylaxis and treatment of deep vein thrombosis (DVT), pulmonary embolism (PE), atrial fibrillation (AF), and myocardial infarction.

MECHANISM OF ACTION

Warfarin is a Vitamin K antagonist which blocks vitamin K from producing active clotting factors in the liver and consequently reduces the number of vitamin-K-dependent clotting factors in your blood. The anticoagulant effect of Warfarin is caused by the inhibition of vitamin K epoxide reductase complex, an enzyme required for activating the vitamin K available in the body. Your blood will then be less likely to form unwanted clots and will inhibit existing clots from growing larger.

WHAT DOES WARFARIN TREAT?

Warfarin is commonly prescribed to:

- prevent and manage venous thromboembolism (blood clots in the veins) and its related medical conditions, deep vein thrombosis (DVT), and pulmonary embolisms (PE).
- prevent and treat thromboembolism in patients suffering from atrial fibrillation
- prevent and treat thromboembolic complications in patients who undergo mechanical heart valve replacement.
- reduce the risk of recurrent myocardial infarction, stroke, systemic embolization after myocardial infarction

It's also prescribed to people with certain health conditions or risks to prevent blood clots from forming in their blood vessels.

WHAT DOES PT/INR STAND FOR?

PT/INR stands for prothrombin time / international normalized ratio and is a calculation based on prothrombin time (PT) results.

Prothrombin is a vitamin K–dependent plasma protein made by the liver. It is also referred to as factor II, one of about 13 active clotting factors in the blood. Clotting factors work together to help stop bleeding after an injury or cut. The test measures how much time it takes for a clot to form in your blood sample and will determine if Warfarin is working the way it should. The target INR range is between 2 and 3. an INR below or above the range can be dangerous for the patient. The dose of warfarin should be adjusted accordingly to bring the target INR back to 2 to 3.

- PT/INR stays within your therapeutic range: your risk of getting a blood clot or bleeding is small.
- PT/INR is below your therapeutic range: your blood is clotting too quickly, putting you at risk for harmful blood clots.
- PT/INR is above your therapeutic range: your blood is clotting too slowly, putting you at risk of bleeding.

DRUG INTERACTIONS AND WARFARIN

Warfarin interacts with many prescriptions and nonprescription medicines (over-the-counter or OTC medicines). The interaction may lower the anticoagulant effect of Warfarin or increase the risk of bleeding. A total of 606 prescriptions and OTC medicines are known to interact with Warfarin. Common medications that can interact with Warfarin include aspirin or aspirin-containing products, acetaminophen (Tylenol), or acetaminophen-containing products, many antibiotics, some cold or allergy medicines, and antacids or laxatives.

You can check warfarin interaction at https://www.drugs.com/drug-interactions/warfarin.html

VITAMIN K AND WARFARIN

Vitamin K is an essential micronutrient the liver needs to produce the vitamin K-dependent coagulation factors required for blood to clot correctly. Vitamin K also plays a critical role in calcium metabolism by activating calcium-bound proteins, which guide calcium to bones and prevent its depositions into arteries, organs, and joint spaces. Without enough vitamin K, the regulation of calcium concentration will be severely affected in various tissues.

On the other hand, the purpose of warfarin therapy is to lower the blood's ability to clot but not prevent it from clotting completely. Increasing your vitamin K intake will interfere with the action of warfarin and substantially decrease its effectiveness.

WHAT IS VITAMIN K?

Vitamin K—the generic name given to a group of fat-soluble vitamins with a similar chemical structure—is naturally present in some foods and available as a dietary supplement. The lactic acid bacteria also produce some vitamin K in our intestines.

Vitamin K exists naturally as phylloquinone (vitamin K1), and a group of menaquinone (vitamin K2)—each of these forms has very different contributions to human health. Vitamin K1 (phylloquinone) is the primary dietary source of vitamin K, accounting for roughly 90% of total vitamin K intake. It is found mainly in green leafy vegetables like spinach, kale, broccoli, green salads, olive oil, and soybean oil.

The most important forms of vitamin K2 are MK-4 and MK-7. Both are found in animal products such as meat, dairy, eggs, cheese, yogurt, liver, natto, butter, egg yolks, and fermented soybeans.

VITAMIN K ALTERS THE BODY'S ABILITY TO METABOLIZE WARFARIN

For most warfarin-treated patients, vitamin K may change how Warfarin works and cause your prothrombin time (PT) test (or INR test) to change. Vitamin K works against Warfarin and lowers your INR values. If you eat more vitamin K, your INR will decrease, showing an alteration of Warfarin's effectiveness. If you eat less vitamin K, your INR will rise, showing that you are at an increased risk of bleeding.

Because vitamin K is essential for your overall health, you don't need to stop eating foods containing vitamin K. Still, you should make informed and more intelligent food choices by focusing on the vitamin k content of foods and try to **keep the amounts from food and supplements about the same every day**.

For this reason, knowing the vitamin K content in all the foods you prefer and knowing how much you can safely eat while keeping your INR in the therapeutic range is essential.

HOW MUCH VITAMIN K DO YOU NEED?

The daily amount of vitamin K you need depends on your age and sex. Recommended Dietary Allowances (RDAs) for vitamin k are listed below in micrograms (mcg).

- for 19+ years old males, the RDA is 120 mcg daily
- for 19+ years old females, the RDA is 90 mcg daily
- for 19+ years old pregnant female, the RDA is 90 mcg daily
- for 19+ years old lactating female, the RDA is 90 mcg daily

PART II
MEAL PLANNING GUIDELINES

MEAL PLANNING GUIDELINES

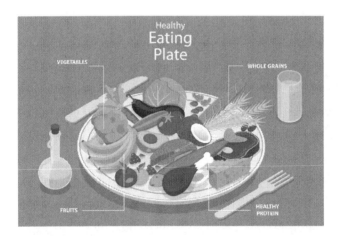

Meal planning allows you to make making informed choices and will work for your personal daily life and tastes. It will ensure that optimal recommendations for a successful Warfarin diet are met. Instead of giving strict recommendations, it gives you options for each food group you can choose.

All foods are assumed to be:

- unprocessed or minimally processed
- in nutrient-dense forms
- lean or low-fat

prepared and cooked with minimal added sugars, salt (sodium), refined carbohydrates, saturated fat, or trans fats.

The total daily calories depend on your personal needs. You have to follow the general guidelines in the next chapters. Recommended amounts of foods in each food group are given to allow you to design your weekly and monthly eating plan.

The five categories of foods are:

- vegetables
- fruits
- grains
- dairy and fortified soy alternatives
- protein foods

GENERAL GUIDELINES

When taking warfarin you must be consistent in how much vitamin K you get daily and aim for stable daily vitamin K intakes. You have to be aware of these guidelines when planning your meals:

1. **aim for a maximum vitamin k (from all sources) in the range of 90-350 mcg per day**.
2. plan regular, balanced meals to avoid high blood sugar levels.
3. **choose healthy cooking methods,** such as broiling, roasting, stir-frying, or grilling.
4. **choose fresh or frozen, unprocessed or canned foods with no added sugar or salt.**
5. **do not eat foods with a vitamin K content greater than**

600% DV per serving size. A recommended DV for adult males equals 120 mcg and for females to 90 mcg.

6. **eat a maximum of 5 servings** (from all sources) **per day of food containing 10%-50% DV of vitamin K.**

7. **eat a maximum of 2½ servings of food** (from all sources) with 50-100% DV of vitamin K.

8. **eat a maximum of 1 serving per day of food** (from all sources) containing 100%-150% DV of vitamin K.

9. **reduce serving sizes for foods with vitamin K content greater than 150% DV** per serving size. If you eat a half-serving size then divide vitamin K content by 2.

10. **choose fresh or frozen, unprocessed,** or canned foods with no added sugar or salt.

11. **exclude trans fats in foods.** Trans fats include margarine, vegetable shortening, French fries, powdered milk, and frozen pizza.

12. **avoid highly processed foods.** Examples of highly processed foods include sugary drinks, flavored potato chips, poultry nuggets and sticks, and fish nuggets.

VEGETABLES AND VEGETABLES PRODUCTS

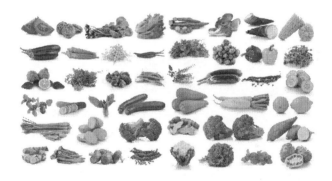

■ WHAT IS THE PORTION SIZE?

The typical serving sizes for vegetables and vegetable juices are equivalent to:

- 1 cup raw or salad vegetables
- ½ cup cooked vegetables
- ¾ cup (6oz) vegetable juice homemade and unsweetened
- ½ cup of cooked beans, lentils, and peas

◼ How Much a Day?

Total vegetable intake: up to 10 servings

Foods listed here have vitamin k content greater than or equal to 60 mcg per serving size, which corresponds to 50% of the recommended daily value. This simplified list aims to increase your awareness of some foods rich in vitamin K. More comprehensive lists and details about serving sizes are provided in part III (Vitamin K Foods Lists)

◼ VEGETABLES CONTAINING 60%-100% DV OF VITAMIN K: THE SIMPLIFIED LIST

Examples of foods include:

- **Asparagus Cooked, From Canned (82.9% DV)**; Serving size = 1 cup, 242 g
- **Broccoli Raw (77.1% DV)**; Serving size = 1 cup chopped , 91 g
- **Broccoli, Raab (74.7% DV)**; Serving size = 1 cup chopped , 40 g
- **Cabbage Common, Cooked Boiled, Drained (67.9% DV)**; Serving size = 1/2 cup, shredded, 75 g
- **Cabbage, Creamed (99.3% DV)**; Serving size = 1 cup , 200 g
- **Carrot Dehydrated (66.6% DV)**; Serving size = 1 cup , 74 g
- **Chicory Greens (71.9% DV)**; Serving size = 1 cup, chopped , 29 g
- **Chinese Broccoli, Cooked, From Fresh or Frozen (61.4% DV)**; Serving size = 1 cup, 88 g
- **Chrysanthemum (72.9% DV)**; Serving size = 1 cup, 25 g
- **Endive (96.3% DV)**; Serving size = 1 head, chopped , 50 g
- **Jute Potherb (molokhia), Cooked Boiled (78.3% DV)**; Serving size = 1 cup, 87 g

- **Luffa, Cooked With Fat (63.9% DV)**; Serving size = 1 cup, 183 g
- **Pea Salad (96.3% DV)**; Serving size = 1 cup , 214 g
- **Pumpkin Leaves, Cooked Boiled, Drained** (63.9% DV); Serving size = 1 cup, 71 g
- **Radicchio (85.1% DV)**; Serving size = 1 cup, shredded , 40 g
- **Savoy Cabbage, Cooked Without Fat (86% DV)**; Serving size = 1 cup, 145 g
- **Sour Pickled Cucumber (60.8% DV)**; Serving size = 1 cup, 155 g
- **Sweet Potato Leaves, Raw (88.2% DV)**; Serving size = 1 cup, chopped, 35 g
- **Watercress (70.8% DV)**; Serving size = 1 cup, chopped , 34 g

---

■ VEGETABLES CONTAINING 100%-200% DV OF VITAMIN K: THE SIMPLIFIED LIST

- **Beet Greens, Raw (126.7% DV)**; Serving size = 1 cup, 38 g
- **Broccoli Fresh or Frozen, Cooked Without Fat (182.3% DV)**; Serving size = 1 cup, fresh, cut stalks, 156 g
- **Broccoli, Cooked Boiled, Drained (183.4% DV)**; Serving size = 1 cup, fresh, cut stalks, 156 g
- **Brussels Sprouts Cooked, From Fresh or Frozen, Without Fat (180.1% DV)**; Serving size = 1 cup, 155 g
- **Brussels Sprouts, Cooked Boiled, Drained (129% DV)**; Serving size = 1/2 cup, 80 g
- **Brussels Sprouts, From Fresh or Frozen, Creamed (148.6% DV)**; Serving size = 1 cup, 228 g
- **Brussels Sprouts, Raw (129.8% DV)**; Serving size = 1 cup, 88 g
- **Cabbage Mustard (123.3% DV)**; Serving size = 1 cup, 128 g

- **Cabbage Salad Or Coleslaw, Made With Various Dressing (average value) (141% DV)**; Serving size = 1 cup, 219 g
- **Chrysanthemum Garland, Cooked Boiled, Drained (118.9% DV)**; Serving size = 1 cup, 100 g
- **Collards (131.2% DV)**; Serving size = 1 cup, chopped, 36 g
- **Escarole, Creamed (183.8% DV)**; Serving size = 1 cup, 200 g
- **Fennel Bulb, Cooked Without Fat (174.3% DV)**; Serving size = 1 fennel bulb, 211 g
- **Green Cabbage, Cooked Without Fat (135% DV)**; Serving size = 1 cup, 150 g
- **Mustard Greens (120.2% DV)**; Serving size = 1 cup, chopped, 56 g
- **New Zealand Spinach (157.3% DV)**; Serving size = 1 cup, chopped, 56 g
- **Poke Greens, Cooked Without Fat (138.6% DV)**; Serving size = 1 cup, 155 g
- **Spinach (120.8% DV)**; Serving size = 1 cup, 30 g
- **Spring Onions (172.5% DV)**; Serving size = 1 cup, chopped, 100 g
- **Turnip Greens (115.1% DV)**; Serving size = 1 cup, chopped, 55 g
- **Turnip Greens With Roots, Cooked, From Canned, Cooked With Fat (187.8% DV)**; Serving size = 1 cup, 168 g

■ VEGETABLES CONTAINING 200%-600% DV OF VITAMIN K: THE SIMPLIFIED LIST

- **Amaranth Leaves, Raw (266% DV)**; Serving size = 1 cup, 28 g
- **Beet Greens, Cooked Boiled, Drained (580.8% DV)**; Serving size = 1 cup, 144 g
- **Beet Greens, Cooked, Without Fat (576.8% DV)**; Serving size = 1 cup, 144 g

- **Broccoli, Raab, Cooked, Without Fat (360.6% DV); Serving size = 1 cup, 170 g**
- **Chamnamul, Cooked, Without Fat (492.7% DV)**; Serving size = 1 cup, 146 g
- **Chard Swiss, Cooked Boiled, Drained** (477.3% DV); Serving size = 1 cup, chopped, 175 g
- **Collards Canned, Cooked Without Fat (542% DV); Serving size = 1 cup, canned, 162 g**
- Cress, Fresh, Frozen Or Canned, Cooked Without Fat (428.2% DV); Serving size = 1 cup, 135 g
- **Dandelion Greens, Cooked Boiled, Drained (314% DV)**; Serving size = 1 cup, chopped, 105 g
- **Escarole, Cooked, Without Fat (227.8% DV)**; Serving size = 1 cup, 130 g
- **Kale (422.1% DV)**; Serving size = 1 cup, chopped, 130 g
- **Onions Green Fresh or Frozen, Cooked Without Fat (393.7% DV)**; Serving size = 1 cup, chopped, 219 g
- **Spinach, Cooked Boiled, Drained (390.8% DV)**; Serving size = 1/2 cup, 95 g
- **Swiss Chard (249% DV)**; Serving size = 1 cup, 36 g
- **Watercress, Cooked, Without Fat (283.7% DV)**; Serving size = 1 cup, 137 g

FRUITS AND FRUITS PRODUCTS

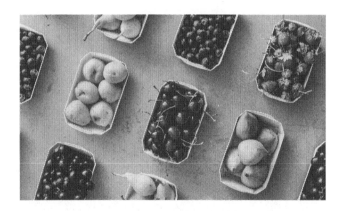

The majority of fruit and vegetables are nutrient-dense, low-calorie, and packed full of essential nutrients such as vitamins, minerals, and fiber.

◼ WHAT IS THE PORTION SIZE?

The typical serving sizes for fruits and fruits juices are equivalent to:

- 1 medium piece

- 1 cup (6 oz) of sliced fruits
- ¾ cup (6 oz) of fruit juice

How Much a Day?

2 to 4 servings per day

■ FRUITS CONTAINING > 50% DV OF VITAMIN K: THE SIMPLIFIED LIST

- **Fruit Salad, Including Citrus Fruits (53.6% DV)**; Serving size = 1 cup, 188 g
- **Kiwifruit (60.4% DV)**; Serving size = 1 cup, sliced, 180 g
- **Plums Dried (53.9% DV)**; Serving size = 1 cup, pitted, 248 g

---

The fruit food group comprises whole fruits and fruit products (100% fruit juice). Whole fruits can be eaten in various forms, such as cut, cubed, sliced, or diced. At least 60% of the recommended amount of total fruit should come from whole fruit rather than 100% juice. Juices should be without added sugars or food additives.

Strategies to increase total fruit intake include

1. often consuming fruits
2. adding fruits to breakfast.
3. choosing more whole fruits as snacks
4. choosing and carrying fruit with you to eat later
5. creating adequate pairings with your favorite foods

■ FRUITS: THE SIMPLIFIED LIST

- **apples** (all fresh, frozen, dried fruits or 100% fruit juices)
- **Asian pears** (all fresh, frozen, dried fruits or 100% fruit juices)
- **bananas** (all fresh, frozen, dried fruits or 100% fruit juices)
- **blackberries** (all fresh, frozen, dried fruits or 100% fruit juices)
- **blueberries** (all fresh, frozen, dried fruits or 100% fruit juices)
- **currants** (all fresh, frozen, dried fruits or 100% fruit juices)
- **huckleberries** (all fresh, frozen, dried fruits or 100% fruit juices)
- **kiwifruit** (all fresh, frozen, dried fruits or 100% fruit juices)
- **mulberries** (all fresh, frozen, dried fruits or 100% fruit juices)
- **raspberries** (all fresh, frozen, dried fruits or 100% fruit juices)
- **strawberries** (all fresh, frozen, dried fruits or 100% fruit juices)
- **calamondin** (all fresh, frozen, dried fruits or 100% fruit juices)
- **grapefruit** (all fresh, frozen, dried fruits or 100% fruit juices)
- **lemons** (all fresh, frozen, dried fruits or 100% fruit juices)
- **limes** (all fresh, frozen, dried fruits or 100% fruit juices)
- **oranges** (all fresh, frozen, dried fruits or 100% fruit juices)
- **pomelos** (all fresh, frozen, dried fruits or 100% fruit juices)
- **cherries** (all fresh, frozen, dried fruits or 100% fruit juices)
- **dates** (all fresh, frozen, dried fruits or 100% fruit juices)
- **figs** (all fresh, frozen, dried fruits or 100% fruit juices)
- **grapes** (all fresh, frozen, dried fruits or 100% fruit juices)
- **guava** (all fresh, frozen, dried fruits or 100% fruit juices)
- **lychee** (all fresh, frozen, dried fruits or 100% fruit juices)
- **mangoes** (all fresh, frozen, dried fruits or 100% fruit juices)
- **nectarines** (all fresh, frozen, dried fruits or 100% fruit juices)
- **peaches** (all fresh, frozen, dried fruits or 100% fruit juices)
- **pears** (all fresh, frozen, dried fruits or 100% fruit juices)
- **plums** (all fresh, frozen, dried fruits or 100% fruit juices)

- **pomegranates** (all fresh, frozen, dried fruits or 100% fruit juices)
- **rhubarb** (all fresh, frozen, dried fruits or 100% fruit juices)
- **sapote** (all fresh, frozen, dried fruits or 100% fruit juices)
- **soursop** (all fresh, frozen, dried fruits or 100% fruit juices)

GRAINS

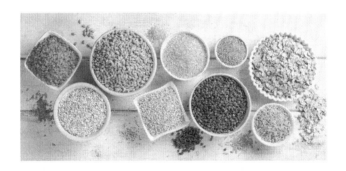

■ WHAT IS THE PORTION SIZE?

The typical serving sizes for cereals and grains are equivalent to:

- ⅓ cup breakfast cereal or muesli
- ½ cup of cooked cereal, or other cooked grain
- ⅓ cup of cooked rice (white rice excluded), and other small grains
- ½ cup of cold cereal

How Much a Day?

Up to 3 servings per day.

■ WHOLE GRAINS: THE SIMPLIFIED LIST

- **barley** (all whole-grain products or used as ingredients)
- **brown rice** (all whole-grain products or used as ingredients)
- **buckwheat** (all whole-grain products or used as ingredients)
- **bulgur** (all whole-grain products or used as ingredients)
- **millet** (all whole-grain products or used as ingredients)
- **oats (Avena sativa L.)** (all whole-grain products or used as ingredients)
- **quinoa** (all whole-grain products or used as ingredients)
- **dark rye** (all whole-grain products or used as ingredients)
- **whole-wheat bread** (all whole-grain products or used as ingredients)
- **whole-wheat chapati** (all whole-grain products or used as ingredients)
- **whole-grain cereals** (all whole-grain products or used as ingredients)
- **wild rice** (all whole-grain products or used as ingredients)

DAIRY AND FORTIFIED SOY ALTERNATIVES

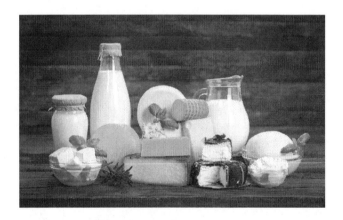

◼ WHAT IS THE PORTION SIZE?

The typical serving sizes for dairy products are equivalent to:

- 1 cup of milk, soy beverage, or yogurt
- ⅓ cup of cottage cheese
- 1 oz of cheese

People with celiac disease or lactose intolerance should consume dairy alternatives

How Much a Day?

Up to 3 servings per day

■ DAIRY AND FORTIFIED SOY ALTERNATIVES: THE SIMPLIFIED LIST

- **buttermilk** (all fluid, evaporated milk, or dry including lactose-free and lactose-reduced products)
- **soy beverages** (all fluid, evaporated milk, or dry including lactose-free and lactose-reduced products)
- **soy milk** (all fluid, evaporated milk, or dry including lactose-free and lactose-reduced products)
- **yogurt** (without added sugar and food additives) (all fluid, evaporated milk, or dry including lactose-free and lactose-reduced products)
- **kefir** (without added sugar and food additives) (all fluid, evaporated milk, or dry including lactose-free and lactose-reduced products)
- **frozen yogurt** (without added sugar and food additives) (all fluid, evaporated milk, or dry including lactose-free and lactose-reduced products)
- **cheeses** (all fluid, evaporated milk, or dry including lactose-free and lactose-reduced products)

PROTEIN FOODS

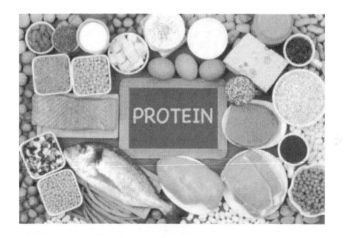

Eating a daily adequate amount of protein is very important for your health. Unlike carbohydrates and fat, your body does not store protein, and you need to eat enough to stay healthy. Animal-based foods are excellent protein sources because they offer a complete composition of essential amino acids with higher bioavailability and digestibility (>90%). Therefore, the main principle to observe here when designing your meal program is to keep a weekly proteins intake equivalent to:

- 30 servings of animal proteins (mainly lean white meat and eggs)
- 10 servings of seafood
- 5 servings of nuts and seeds

■ MEATS CONTAINING > 50% DV OF VITAMIN K: THE SIMPLIFIED LIST

- **Beef, Liver Braised (65.2% DV)**; Serving size = 3 oz, 85 g
- **Bockwurst Pork Veal, Raw (53.3% DV)**; Serving size = 1 sausage, 91 g
- **Ham, Or Pork Salad (67.2% DV)**; Serving size = 1 cup, 182 g
- **Veal, Cordon Bleu (53.6% DV)**; Serving size = 1 roll, 229 g

---

■ MEATS, POULTRY, EGGS, SEAFOODS: WHAT IS THE PORTION SIZE?

The typical serving sizes for the "meats, poultry, eggs", "seafood", and "nuts, seeds, soy Products" groups are equivalent to:

- 3 to 4 ounces of cooked, baked, or broiled beef
- 3 to 4 ounces of cooked, baked, or broiled veal
- 3 to 4 ounces of cooked, baked, or broiled poultry
- 3 to 4 ounces of cooked or canned fish
- 3 to 4 ounces of seafood
- 2 medium eggs
- ⅓ cup of nuts (5 large or 10 small nuts)
- 2 tablespoons of nut butter
- 2 tablespoons of nut spread

▣ Meats, Poultry, Eggs: The simplified List

Meats (lean or low-fats) include:

- beef, goat, lamb, and pork (fat red meats must be limited due to their pro-inflammatory effects). You have to choose lean meats preferably grass-fed beef, lamb, or bison
- game meat (e.g., bison, moose, elk, deer)

Poultry (lean or low-fats) includes

- chicken
- turkey
- cornish hens
- duck
- game birds (e.g., ostrich, pheasant, and quail)
- goose.

Eggs include

- chicken eggs
- turkey eggs
- duck eggs and other birds' eggs

▣ Seafood: The simplified List

Seafood include

- salmon
- sardine
- anchovy

- black sea bass
- catfish
- clams
- cod
- crab
- crawfish
- flounder
- haddock
- hake
- herring
- lobster
- mullet
- oyster
- perch
- pollock
- scallop
- shrimp
- sole
- squid
- tilapia
- freshwater trout
- tuna

■ NUTS, SEEDS, SOY PRODUCTS: THE SIMPLIFIED LIST

Nuts (and nut butter) include

- almonds
- pecans
- Brazil nuts
- pistachios
- hazelnuts
- macadamias

- pine nuts
- walnuts
- cashew nuts

Seeds (and seed butter) include:

- pumpkin seeds
- psyllium seeds
- chia seeds.
- flax seeds
- sunflower seeds
- sesame seeds
- poppy seeds

PART III
VITAMIN K FOODS LISTS

The classification of foods may vary between books, thus the essential factor to consider is the serving size. Data is based on the USDA National Nutrient Database, which is the most authoritative source of food composition data in the United States.

ESSENTIAL THINGS TO REMEMBER:

– Serving size is a crucial factor in your warfarin diet. Pay attention to serving sizes. Eating more than one serving of moderate vitamin K food may equal one high vitamin K food.

Be consistent and maintain your vitamin K intake about the same each day.

ABBREVIATIONS

- dia diameter
- DV daily value: the DV for vitamin K is 120 mcg for adults and children aged 4 years and older
- fl oz fluid ounce
- g gram
- kcal kilocalorie (commonly known as calories)
- IU International Units
- lb pound
- mcg microgram
- mg milligram
- ml milliliter
- oz ounce
- pkg package
- RE retinol equivalent
- sq square
- tbsp tablespoon
- tsp teaspoon
- Tr trace
- tsp teaspoon

BAKED PRODUCTS

Air Filled Fritter ☞ Vitamin K = 13.5 mcg; DV = 11.3%; Serving size: 1 turnover, 57 g

Apple Strudel ☞ Vitamin K = 0.8 mcg; DV = 0.7%; Serving size: 1 oz, 28.4 g

Arepa Dominicana ☞ Vitamin K = 3.8 mcg; DV = 3.2%; Serving size: 1 piece, 115 g

Bagel—(Oat Bran) ☞ Vitamin K = 0.1 mcg; DV = 0.1%; Serving size: 1 mini bagel, 26 g

Bagel—Multigrain ☞ Vitamin K = 0.4 mcg; DV = 0.3%; Serving size: 1 miniature, 26 g

Bagel—Oat Bran ☞ Vitamin K = 0.4 mcg; DV = 0.3%; Serving size: 1 miniature, 26 g

Bagel—Pumpernickel ☞ Vitamin K = 0.4 mcg; DV = 0.3%; Serving size: 1 miniature, 26 g

Bagel—Wheat ☞ Vitamin K = 1.5 mcg; DV = 1.3%; Serving size: 1 bagel, 98 g

Bagel—Whole Grain White ☛ Vitamin K = 0.4 mcg; DV = 0.3%; Serving size: 1 miniature, 26 g

Bagel—Whole Wheat ☛ Vitamin K = 0.4 mcg; DV = 0.3%; Serving size: 1 miniature, 26 g

Baklava ☛ Vitamin K = 2.7 mcg; DV = 2.3%; Serving size: 1 piece, 78 g

Basbousa ☛ Vitamin K = 3.4 mcg; DV = 2.8%; Serving size: 1 piece, 82 g

Biscuit Cheese ☛ Vitamin K = 1.2 mcg; DV = 1%; Serving size: 1 biscuit (2" dia), 30 g

Biscuit Cinnamon-Raisin ☛ Vitamin K = 4.5 mcg; DV = 3.8%; Serving size: 1 biscuit (3" dia), 64 g

Biscuit Whole Wheat ☛ Vitamin K = 0.9 mcg; DV = 0.8%; Serving size: 1 small (1-1/2" dia), 14 g

Blueberry Pie ☛ Vitamin K = 3 mcg; DV = 2.5%; Serving size: 1 oz, 28.4 g

Bread— Chapati ☛ Vitamin K = 1.4 mcg; DV = 1.2%; Serving size: 1 piece, 43 g

Bread—Barley ☛ Vitamin K = 1.2 mcg; DV = 1%; Serving size: 1 small or thin/very thin slice, 22 g

Bread—Caressed Puerto Rican Style ☛ Vitamin K = 0.4 mcg; DV = 0.3%; Serving size: 1 slice, 25 g

Bread—Cinnamon ☛ Vitamin K = 2.7 mcg; DV = 2.3%; Serving size: 1 slice 1 serving, 28 g

Bread—French Or Vienna ☛ Vitamin K = 0.3 mcg; DV = 0.3%; Serving size: 1 slice 1 serving, 48 g

Bread—Italian ☛ Vitamin K = 0.9 mcg; DV = 0.8%; Serving size: 1 oz, 28.4 g

Bread—Multi-Grain ☞ Vitamin K = 0.4 mcg; DV = 0.3%; Serving size: 1 oz, 28.4 g

Bread—Naan Whole Wheat ☞ Vitamin K = 3.5 mcg; DV = 2.9%; Serving size: 1 piece, 106 g

Bread—Nut ☞ Vitamin K = 7.5 mcg; DV = 6.3%; Serving size: 1 slice, 49 g

Bread—Oat Bran ☞ Vitamin K = 0.3 mcg; DV = 0.3%; Serving size: 1 oz, 28.4 g

Bread—Oatmeal ☞ Vitamin K = 0.4 mcg; DV = 0.3%; Serving size: 1 oz, 28.4 g

Bread—Pumpernickel ☞ Vitamin K = 0.2 mcg; DV = 0.2%; Serving size: 1 oz, 28.4 g

Bread—Pumpkin ☞ Vitamin K = 10 mcg; DV = 8.3%; Serving size: 1 slice, 60 g

Bread—Puri Wheat ☞ Vitamin K = 10.2 mcg; DV = 8.5%; Serving size: 1 puri (4-4/5" dia), 36 g

Bread—Rice Bran ☞ Vitamin K = 0.3 mcg; DV = 0.3%; Serving size: 1 oz, 28.4 g

Bread—Roll Mexican Bollilo ☞ Vitamin K = 10.7 mcg; DV = 8.9%; Serving size: 1 piece, 98 g

Bread—White Wheat ☞ Vitamin K = 2.2 mcg; DV = 1.8%; Serving size: 1 slice, 28 g

Bread—Zucchini ☞ Vitamin K = 5.6 mcg; DV = 4.7%; Serving size: 1 slice, 40 g

Brioche ☞ Vitamin K = 1.8 mcg; DV = 1.5%; Serving size: 1 piece, 77 g

Cake Or CupCake—Applesauce ☞ Vitamin K = 10.4 mcg; DV = 8.7%; Serving size: 1 regular cupcake, 75 g

Cake, Or CupCake—Banana ☛ Vitamin K = 12.8 mcg; DV = 10.7%; Serving size: 1 regular cupcake, 75 g

Cake, Or CupCake—Carrot ☛ Vitamin K = 15 mcg; DV = 12.5%; Serving size: 1 regular cupcake, 75 g

Cake, Or CupCake—German Chocolate ☛ Vitamin K = 20 mcg; DV = 16.7%; Serving size: 1 regular cupcake, 75 g

Cake, Or CupCake—Marble ☛ Vitamin K = 12 mcg; DV = 10%; Serving size: 1 regular cupcake, 75 g

Cake, Or CupCake—Nut ☛ Vitamin K = 7.4 mcg; DV = 6.2%; Serving size: 1 regular cupcake, 75 g

Cake, Or CupCake—Oatmeal ☛ Vitamin K = 4.4 mcg; DV = 3.7%; Serving size: 1 regular cupcake, 50 g

Cake, Or CupCake—Peanut Butter ☛ Vitamin K = 3.6 mcg; DV = 3%; Serving size: 1 regular cupcake, 50 g

Cake, Or CupCake—Pumpkin With Icing Or Filling ☛ Vitamin K = 15 mcg; DV = 12.5%; Serving size: 1 regular cupcake, 75 g

Cake—Snack Cakes Creme-Filled Sponge ☛ Vitamin K = 2.8 mcg; DV = 2.3%; Serving size: 1 oz, 28.4 g

Cake—Sponge—Commercially Prepared, ☛ Vitamin K = 0.1 mcg; DV = 0.1%; Serving size: 1 oz, 28.4 g

Casabe Cassava Bread ☛ Vitamin K = 3.6 mcg; DV = 3%; Serving size: 1 piece (6" dia), 100 g

Cheese Croissants ☛ Vitamin K = 3.1 mcg; DV = 2.6%; Serving size: 1 oz, 28.4 g

Cheese Pastry—Puffs ☛ Vitamin K = 0.8 mcg; DV = 0.7%; Serving size: 1 puff or cheese straw (5" long), 6 g

CheeseCake—Commercially Prepared ☛ Vitamin K = 1.2 mcg; DV = 1%; Serving size: 1 oz, 28.4 g

Chocolate Cake—With Frosting ☞ Vitamin K = 39.9 mcg; DV = 33.3%; Serving size: 1 piece (1/12 of a cake), 138 g

Chocolate Coated Graham Crackers ☞ Vitamin K = 1.7 mcg; DV = 1.4%; Serving size: 3 pieces, 27 g

Churros ☞ Vitamin K = 3.9 mcg; DV = 3.3%; Serving size: 1 churro, 26 g

Cobbler—Apple ☞ Vitamin K = 6.5 mcg; DV = 5.4%; Serving size: 1 cup, 217 g

Cobbler—Apricot ☞ Vitamin K = 9.5 mcg; DV = 7.9%; Serving size: 1 cup, 217 g

Cobbler—Berry ☞ Vitamin K = 29.3 mcg; DV = 24.4%; Serving size: 1 cup, 217 g

Cobbler—Pear ☞ Vitamin K = 11.3 mcg; DV = 9.4%; Serving size: 1 cup, 217 g

Cobbler—Pineapple ☞ Vitamin K = 5.2 mcg; DV = 4.3%; Serving size: 1 cup, 217 g

Cobbler—Rhubarb ☞ Vitamin K = 42.3 mcg; DV = 35.3%; Serving size: 1 cup, 217 g

Cookies—Brownie ☞ Vitamin K = 1.3 mcg; DV = 1.1%; Serving size: 1 small, 40 g

Cookies—Chocolate Chip ☞ Vitamin K = 0.1 mcg; DV = 0.1%; Serving size: 1 miniature/bite size, 5 g

Cookies—Oatmeal With Chocolate Chips ☞ Vitamin K = 0.4 mcg; DV = 0.3%; Serving size: 1 miniature/bite size, 5 g

Cookies—Brownies ☞ Vitamin K = 1.8 mcg; DV = 1.5%; Serving size: 1 oz, 28.4 g

Cookies—Chocolate Chip Sandwich ☞ Vitamin K = 1.4 mcg; DV = 1.2%; Serving size: 1 cookie, 34 g

Cookies—Chocolate Made With Rice Cereal ☛ Vitamin K = 2.5 mcg; DV = 2.1%; Serving size: 1 cookie, 62 g

Cookies—Oatmeal Sandwich With Creme Filling ☛ Vitamin K = 2.1 mcg; DV = 1.8%; Serving size: 1 cookie 1 serving, 38 g

Cookies—Raisin Soft-Type ☛ Vitamin K = 1.1 mcg; DV = 0.9%; Serving size: 1 oz, 28.4 g

Corn Muffins ☛ Vitamin K = 0.7 mcg; DV = 0.6%; Serving size: 1 oz, 28.4 g

Corn Pone Baked ☛ Vitamin K = 6.8 mcg; DV = 5.7%; Serving size: 1 pone, 377 g

Corn Pone Fried ☛ Vitamin K = 2.9 mcg; DV = 2.4%; Serving size: 1 piece, 61 g

Cracker Meal ☛ Vitamin K = 0.1 mcg; DV = 0.1%; Serving size: 1 oz, 28.4 g

Crackers—Cheese Regular ☛ Vitamin K = 1.3 mcg; DV = 1.1%; Serving size: 1/2 oz, 14.2 g

Crackers—Cheese Sandwich-Type With Cheese Filling ☛ Vitamin K = 8 mcg; DV = 6.7%; Serving size: 6 cracker 1 cracker = 6.5g, 39 g

Crackers—Multigrain ☛ Vitamin K = 5 mcg; DV = 4.2%; Serving size: 4 crackers, 14 g

Crackers—Rye Wafers Plain ☛ Vitamin K = 0.8 mcg; DV = 0.7%; Serving size: 1/2 oz, 14.2 g

Crackers—Standard Snack-Type Regular ☛ Vitamin K = 11.1 mcg; DV = 9.3%; Serving size: 5 crackers, 16 g

Crackers—Whole-Wheat ☛ Vitamin K = 7.6 mcg; DV = 6.3%; Serving size: 1 serving, 28 g

Cream Puff Eclair Custard ☛ Vitamin K = 7.6 mcg; DV = 6.3%; Serving size: 4 oz, 113 g

Cream Puff Shell ☛ Vitamin K = 7 mcg; DV = 5.8%; Serving size: 1 oz, 28.4 g

Crisp Blueberry ☛ Vitamin K = 58.3 mcg; DV = 48.6%; Serving size: 1 cup, 246 g

Crisp Cherry ☛ Vitamin K = 23.1 mcg; DV = 19.3%; Serving size: 1 cup, 246 g

Crisp Peach ☛ Vitamin K = 23.1 mcg; DV = 19.3%; Serving size: 1 cup, 246 g

Crisp Rhubarb ☛ Vitamin K = 53.1 mcg; DV = 44.3%; Serving size: 1 cup, 246 g

Croutons Seasoned ☛ Vitamin K = 1.1 mcg; DV = 0.9%; Serving size: 1/2 oz, 14.2 g

Crumpet ☛ Vitamin K = 0.2 mcg; DV = 0.2%; Serving size: 1 small, 20 g

Danish Pastry—Cheese ☛ Vitamin K = 2 mcg; DV = 1.7%; Serving size: 1 oz, 28.4 g

Doughnuts—Chocolate Raised Or Yeast ☛ Vitamin K = 5.6 mcg; DV = 4.7%; Serving size: 1 doughnut (3" dia), 50 g

Doughnuts—Custard-Filled With Icing ☛ Vitamin K = 4.8 mcg; DV = 4%; Serving size: 1 doughnut, 70 g

Doughnuts—French Crullers Glazed ☛ Vitamin K = 2.3 mcg; DV = 1.9%; Serving size: 1 oz, 28.4 g

Dumpling Plain ☛ Vitamin K = 0.3 mcg; DV = 0.3%; Serving size: 1 small, 18 g

Empanada Mexican Turnover Fruit-Filled ☛ Vitamin K = 9.9 mcg; DV = 8.3%; Serving size: 1 cup, 142 g

Fig Bars ☛ Vitamin K = 1.6 mcg; DV = 1.3%; Serving size: 1 oz, 28.4 g

Fritter—Apple ☛ Vitamin K = 2 mcg; DV = 1.7%; Serving size: 1 fritter, 17 g

Fritter—Banana ☛ Vitamin K = 3.9 mcg; DV = 3.3%; Serving size: 1 fritter (2" long), 34 g

Fritter—Berry ☛ Vitamin K = 5.2 mcg; DV = 4.3%; Serving size: 1 fritter (1-1/4" dia), 24 g

Garlic Bread ☛ Vitamin K = 10.9 mcg; DV = 9.1%; Serving size: 1 small slice, 37 g

Gingersnaps ☛ Vitamin K = 0.7 mcg; DV = 0.6%; Serving size: 1 oz, 28.4 g

Hush Puppies ☛ Vitamin K = 6.7 mcg; DV = 5.6%; Serving size: 1 oz, 28.4 g

Muffin English Oat Bran ☛ Vitamin K = 1 mcg; DV = 0.8%; Serving size: 1 muffin, 58 g

Muffin English Wheat Bran ☛ Vitamin K = 0.6 mcg; DV = 0.5%; Serving size: 1 muffin, 58 g

Muffin—Whole Grain ☛ Vitamin K = 4.5 mcg; DV = 3.8%; Serving size: 1 miniature, 25 g

Muffins Blueberry Toaster-Type ☛ Vitamin K = 5.5 mcg; DV = 4.6%; Serving size: 1 oz, 28.4 g

Muffins Blueberry—Commercially Prepared ☛ Vitamin K = 11.1 mcg; DV = 9.3%; Serving size: 1 oz, 28.4 g

Muffins Oat Bran ☛ Vitamin K = 3.7 mcg; DV = 3.1%; Serving size: 1 oz, 28.4 g

Pancakes—Plain Frozen ☛ Vitamin K = 2.1 mcg; DV = 1.8%; Serving size: 1 oz, 28.4 g

Pannetone ☛ Vitamin K = 0.2 mcg; DV = 0.2%; Serving size: 1 slice, 27 g

Pastry—Cheese-Filled ☞ Vitamin K = 3.8 mcg; DV = 3.2%; Serving size: 1 pastry, 28 g

Pastry—Cookies—Type Fried ☞ Vitamin K = 8.7 mcg; DV = 7.3%; Serving size: 1 pastry, 46 g

Pastry—Fruit-Filled ☞ Vitamin K = 13.7 mcg; DV = 11.4%; Serving size: 1 pastry, 78 g

Pie Crust—Cookie-Type Chocolate ☞ Vitamin K = 33.1 mcg; DV = 27.6%; Serving size: 1 crust, 182 g

Pie Crust—Cookie-Type Graham Cracker ☞ Vitamin K = 6.2 mcg; DV = 5.2%; Serving size: 1 oz, 28.4 g

Pie Crust—Cookie-Type—Graham Cracker Chilled ☞ Vitamin K = 7.3 mcg; DV = 6.1%; Serving size: 1 piece, 30 g

Pie Crust—Standard-Type—Prepared From Recipe ☞ Vitamin K = 3.4 mcg; DV = 2.8%; Serving size: 1 piece, 23 g

Pie Tofu With Fruit ☞ Vitamin K = 18.4 mcg; DV = 15.3%; Serving size: 1/8 pie (9" dia), 144 g

Pie—Apple Diet ☞ Vitamin K = 1.6 mcg; DV = 1.3%; Serving size: 1 individual serving, 85 g

Pie—Banana Cream ☞ Vitamin K = 5.9 mcg; DV = 4.9%; Serving size: 1 tart, 117 g

Pie—Banana Cream ☞ Vitamin K = 1.8 mcg; DV = 1.5%; Serving size: 1 oz, 28.4 g

Pie—Blackberry Individual Size Or Tart ☞ Vitamin K = 19.9 mcg; DV = 16.6%; Serving size: 1 tart, 117 g

Pie—Blueberry Individual Size Or Tart ☞ Vitamin K = 19.8 mcg; DV = 16.5%; Serving size: 1 tart, 117 g

Pie—Buttermilk ☞ Vitamin K = 12.7 mcg; DV = 10.6%; Serving size: 1/8 pie (9" dia), 144 g

Pie—Cherry—Commercially Prepared, ☛ Vitamin K = 2.2 mcg; DV = 1.8%; Serving size: 1 oz, 28.4 g

Pie—Chocolate Crème ☛ Vitamin K = 11.4 mcg; DV = 9.5%; Serving size: 1 serving .167 pie, 120 g

Pie—Coconut Cream ☛ Vitamin K = 5.5 mcg; DV = 4.6%; Serving size: 1 tart, 117 g

Pie—Custard ☛ Vitamin K = 2 mcg; DV = 1.7%; Serving size: 1 tart, 117 g

Pie—Lemon Cream ☛ Vitamin K = 10.1 mcg; DV = 8.4%; Serving size: 1/8 pie (9" dia), 144 g

Pie—Peach ☛ Vitamin K = 10.1 mcg; DV = 8.4%; Serving size: 1 tart, 117 g

Pie—Pear ☛ Vitamin K = 10.8 mcg; DV = 9%; Serving size: 1 tart, 117 g

Pie—Pecan ☛ Vitamin K = 4.4 mcg; DV = 3.7%; Serving size: 1 oz, 28.4 g

Pie—Pumpkin ☛ Vitamin K = 3.7 mcg; DV = 3.1%; Serving size: 1 oz, 28.4 g

Pie—Raisin ☛ Vitamin K = 8.9 mcg; DV = 7.4%; Serving size: 1 tart, 117 g

Pie—Raspberry Cream ☛ Vitamin K = 9.5 mcg; DV = 7.9%; Serving size: 1/8 pie (9" dia), 144 g

Pie—Rhubarb ☛ Vitamin K = 22.8 mcg; DV = 19%; Serving size: 1 tart, 117 g

Pie—Squash ☛ Vitamin K = 5.9 mcg; DV = 4.9%; Serving size: 1/8 pie (9" dia), 154 g

Pie—Strawberry Cream ☛ Vitamin K = 6.9 mcg; DV = 5.8%; Serving size: 1/8 pie (10" dia), 181 g

Pie—Sweet Potato ☞ Vitamin K = 7.4 mcg; DV = 6.2%; Serving size: 1/8 pie (10" dia), 191 g

Pie—Vanilla Cream ☞ Vitamin K = 1.9 mcg; DV = 1.6%; Serving size: 1 oz, 28.4 g

Pie—Yogurt Frozen ☞ Vitamin K = 15 mcg; DV = 12.5%; Serving size: 1/8 pie (9" dia), 144 g

Plain Graham Crackers ☞ Vitamin K = 4.1 mcg; DV = 3.4%; Serving size: 1 oz, 28.4 g

Puff Pastry ☞ Vitamin K = 4.6 mcg; DV = 3.8%; Serving size: 1 oz, 28.4 g

Roll Cheese ☞ Vitamin K = 4.2 mcg; DV = 3.5%; Serving size: 1 roll, 41 g

Rolls—Dinner Rye ☞ Vitamin K = 1.3 mcg; DV = 1.1%; Serving size: 1 large, 43 g

Rolls—Dinner Wheat ☞ Vitamin K = 0.8 mcg; DV = 0.7%; Serving size: 1 roll (1 oz), 28 g

Rolls—French ☞ Vitamin K = 0.5 mcg; DV = 0.4%; Serving size: 1 oz, 28.4 g

Rolls—Hamburger Or Hot Dog Wheat ☞ Vitamin K = 3.5 mcg; DV = 2.9%; Serving size: 1 roll, 51 g

Rolls—Hamburger Or Hotdog Mixed-Grain ☞ Vitamin K = 1.7 mcg; DV = 1.4%; Serving size: 1 roll, 56 g

Rolls—Hamburger Or Hotdog Plain ☞ Vitamin K = 2.1 mcg; DV = 1.8%; Serving size: 1 roll 1 serving, 44 g

Scone ☞ Vitamin K = 4.2 mcg; DV = 3.5%; Serving size: 1 scone, 42 g

Scone With Fruit ☞ Vitamin K = 4 mcg; DV = 3.3%; Serving size: 1 scone, 42 g

Sopaipilla ☛ Vitamin K = 1.1 mcg; DV = 0.9%; Serving size: 1 sopaipilla, 12 g

Strudel—Cheese ☛ Vitamin K = 3.5 mcg; DV = 2.9%; Serving size: 1 piece, 64 g

Strudel—Cherry ☛ Vitamin K = 4.2 mcg; DV = 3.5%; Serving size: 1 piece, 64 g

Strudel—Peach ☛ Vitamin K = 4.6 mcg; DV = 3.8%; Serving size: 1 piece, 64 g

Strudel—Pineapple ☛ Vitamin K = 4 mcg; DV = 3.3%; Serving size: 1 piece, 64 g

Taco Shells Baked ☛ Vitamin K = 1.1 mcg; DV = 0.9%; Serving size: 1 shell, 12.9 g

Tamale Sweet ☛ Vitamin K = 2.2 mcg; DV = 1.8%; Serving size: 1 tamale, 34 g

Tiramisu ☛ Vitamin K = 3 mcg; DV = 2.5%; Serving size: 1 piece, 174 g

Toaster Pastries Fruit (With Apple Blueberry Cherry Strawberry) ☛ Vitamin K = 4.4 mcg; DV = 3.7%; Serving size: 1 oz, 28.4 g

Tortillas—Ready-To-Bake ☛ Vitamin K = 3.5 mcg; DV = 2.9%; Serving size: 1 tortilla, 48 g

Turnover Or Dumpling Apple ☛ Vitamin K = 8.1 mcg; DV = 6.8%; Serving size: 1 turnover, 82 g

Turnover Or Dumpling Berry ☛ Vitamin K = 13.3 mcg; DV = 11.1%; Serving size: 1 turnover, 78 g

Turnover Or Dumpling Cherry ☛ Vitamin K = 7 mcg; DV = 5.8%; Serving size: 1 turnover, 78 g

Turnover Or Dumpling Lemon ☛ Vitamin K = 6.5 mcg; DV = 5.4%; Serving size: 1 turnover, 78 g

Turnover Or Dumpling Peach ☛ Vitamin K = 7.6 mcg; DV = 6.3%; Serving size: 1 turnover, 78 g

Waffles—Buttermilk Frozen ☛ Vitamin K = 4.1 mcg; DV = 3.4%; Serving size: 1 waffle, square, 39 g

Waffles—Chocolate Chip Frozen ☛ Vitamin K = 6.5 mcg; DV = 5.4%; Serving size: 2 waffles, 70 g

Waffles—Plain Frozen ☛ Vitamin K = 2.2 mcg; DV = 1.8%; Serving size: 1 oz, 28.4 g

White Pizza—Cheese Thick Crust ☛ Vitamin K = 5.5 mcg; DV = 4.6%; Serving size: 1 piece, 141 g

White Pizza—Cheese Thin Crust ☛ Vitamin K = 4.1 mcg; DV = 3.4%; Serving size: 1 piece, 92 g

Yam Buns; Puerto Rican Style ☛ Vitamin K = 34.9 mcg; DV = 29.1%; Serving size: 1 cup, 153 g

BEANS AND LENTILS

Beans—Baked Canned, Cooked without Fat ☛ Vitamin K = 2.6 mcg; DV= 2.2%; Serving size: 1 cup, 259 g

Beans—Black Turtle Mature Seeds Canned, Cooked without Fat ☛ Vitamin K = 5.5 mcg; DV= 4.6%; Serving size: 1 cup, 240 g

Beans—Dry, Cooked With Meat ☛ Vitamin K = 26.1 mcg; DV= 21.8%; Serving size: 1 cup, 266 g

Beans—Great Northern Mature Seeds Canned, Cooked without Fat ☛ Vitamin K = 7.9 mcg; DV= 6.6%; Serving size: 1 cup, 262 g

Beans—Kidney Red Mature Seeds Canned, Cooked without Fat ☛ Vitamin K = 9 mcg; DV= 7.5%; Serving size: 1 cup rinsed solids, 158 g

Beans—Pinto Mature Seeds Canned, Cooked without Fat ☛ Vitamin K = 5 mcg; DV= 4.2%; Serving size: 1 cup, 240 g

Beans—White Mature Seeds Canned, Cooked without Fat ☛ Vitamin K = 7.6 mcg; DV= 6.3%; Serving size: 1 cup, 262 g

Black Bean Salad ☛ Vitamin K = 27.3 mcg; DV= 22.8%; Serving size: 1 cup, 231 g

Black Beans ☛ Vitamin K = 5.7 mcg; DV= 4.8%; Serving size: 1 cup, 172 g

Black Beans—Cuban Style ☛ Vitamin K = 11.9 mcg; DV= 9.9%; Serving size: 1 cup, 270 g

Black Brown Or Bayo Beans—Canned, Cooked without Fat ☛ Vitamin K = 5.8 mcg; DV= 4.8%; Serving size: 1 cup, 180 g

Black Brown Or Bayo Beans—Canned Drained, Prepared With Oil or Margarine ☛ Vitamin K = 19.1 mcg; DV= 15.9%; Serving size: 1 cup, 180 g

Black Brown Or Bayo Beans—Dry, Cooked, Cooked without Fat ☛ Vitamin K = 5.9 mcg; DV= 4.9%; Serving size: 1 cup, 180 g

Black Brown Or Bayo Beans—Dry, Cooked Made With Oil ☛ Vitamin K = 20.9 mcg; DV= 17.4%; Serving size: 1 cup, 180 g

Black Turtle Beans ☛ Vitamin K = 6.1 mcg; DV= 5.1%; Serving size: 1 cup, 185 g

Broad Beans—(Fava) ☛ Vitamin K = 4.9 mcg; DV= 4.1%; Serving size: 1 cup, 170 g

Chickpea Flour (Besan) ☛ Vitamin K = 8.4 mcg; DV= 7%; Serving size: 1 cup, 92 g

Chickpeas—Canned Drained, Cooked without Fat ☛ Vitamin K = 6.7 mcg; DV= 5.6%; Serving size: 1 cup, 180 g

Chickpeas—Canned Drained, Prepared With Oil or Margarine ☛ Vitamin K = 21.1 mcg; DV= 17.6%; Serving size: 1 cup, 180 g

Chickpeas—Dry, Cooked, Cooked without Fat ☛ Vitamin K = 7.2 mcg; DV= 6%; Serving size: 1 cup, 180 g

CowPeas—Dry, Cooked, Cooked with Fat ☛ Vitamin K = 18.4 mcg; DV= 15.3%; Serving size: 1 cup, 180 g

CowPeas—Dry, Cooked, Cooked without Fat ☛ Vitamin K = 3.1 mcg; DV= 2.6%; Serving size: 1 cup, 180 g

Edamame ☛ Vitamin K = 41.4 mcg; DV= 34.5%; Serving size: 1 cup, 155 g

Fava Beans—Canned Drained, Prepared With Oil or Margarine ☛ Vitamin K = 19.6 mcg; DV= 16.3%; Serving size: 1 cup, 180 g

Fava Beans—Dry, Cooked, Cooked without Fat ☛ Vitamin K = 5.2 mcg; DV= 4.3%; Serving size: 1 cup, 180 g

Firm Tofu ☛ Vitamin K = 3 mcg; DV= 2.5%; Serving size: 1/2 cup, 126 g

Green Or Yellow Split Peas—Dry, Cooked, Cooked without Fat ☛ Vitamin K = 9 mcg; DV= 7.5%; Serving size: 1 cup, 180 g

Green Or Yellow Split Peas—Dry, Cooked With Oil or Margarine ☛ Vitamin K = 22.1 mcg; DV= 18.4%; Serving size: 1 cup, 180 g

Hummus (Commercial) ☛ Vitamin K = 3.4 mcg; DV= 2.8%; Serving size: 1 tbsp, 15 g

Hummus (Homemade) ☛ Vitamin K = 0.5 mcg; DV= 0.4%; Serving size: 1 tablespoon, 15 g

Kidney Beans ☛ Vitamin K = 14.9 mcg; DV= 12.4%; Serving size: 1 cup, 177 g

Lentils Dry, Cooked, Cooked without Fat ☛ Vitamin K = 3.1 mcg; DV= 2.6%; Serving size: 1 cup, 180 g

Lentils Dry, Cooked Made With Oil or Margarine ☛ Vitamin K = 16.4 mcg; DV= 13.7%; Serving size: 1 cup, 180 g

Lima Beans—Dry, Cooked, Cooked without Fat ☛ Vitamin K = 3.6 mcg; DV= 3%; Serving size: 1 cup, 180 g

Lima Beans—Dry, Cooked Made With Oil or Margarine ☛ Vitamin K = 17.6 mcg; DV= 14.7%; Serving size: 1 cup, 180 g

Miso ☛ Vitamin K = 5 mcg; DV= 4.2%; Serving size: 1 tbsp, 17 g

Mung Beans—Dry, Cooked, Cooked with Fat ☛ Vitamin K = 17.8 mcg; DV= 14.8%; Serving size: 1 cup, 180 g

Mung Beans—Dry, Cooked, Cooked without Fat ☛ Vitamin K = 4.9 mcg; DV= 4.1%; Serving size: 1 cup, 180 g

Natto ☛ Vitamin K = 40.4 mcg; DV= 33.7%; Serving size: 1 cup, 175 g

Peanut—Butter ☛ Vitamin K = 0.2 mcg; DV= 0.2%; Serving size: 2 tbsp, 32 g

Pink Beans—Canned Drained, Prepared With Oil or Margarine ☛ Vitamin K = 21.1 mcg; DV= 17.6%; Serving size: 1 cup, 180 g

Pink Beans—Canned Drained, Cooked without Fat ☛ Vitamin K = 6.7 mcg; DV= 5.6%; Serving size: 1 cup, 180 g

Pink Beans—Dry, Cooked, Cooked with Fat ☛ Vitamin K = 22 mcg; DV= 18.3%; Serving size: 1 cup, 180 g

Pink Beans—Dry, Cooked, Cooked without Fat ☛ Vitamin K = 6.7 mcg; DV= 5.6%; Serving size: 1 cup, 180 g

Pinto Beans—Canned Drained, Cooked without Fat ☛ Vitamin K = 6.3 mcg; DV= 5.3%; Serving size: 1 cup, 180 g

Pinto Beans—Canned Drained, Prepared With Oil or Margarine ☛ Vitamin K = 19.3 mcg; DV= 16.1%; Serving size: 1 cup, 180 g

Pinto Beans—Dry, Cooked, Cooked without Fat ☛ Vitamin K = 6.3 mcg; DV= 5.3%; Serving size: 1 cup, 180 g

Pinto Beans—Dry, Cooked Made With Oil ☛ Vitamin K = 21.4 mcg; DV= 17.8%; Serving size: 1 cup, 180 g

Red Kidney Beans—Canned Drained, Cooked without Fat ☛ Vitamin K = 12.2 mcg; DV= 10.2%; Serving size: 1 cup, 180 g

Red Kidney Beans—Canned Drained, Prepared With Oil or

Margarine ☛ Vitamin K = 26.3 mcg; DV= 21.9%; Serving size: 1 cup, 180 g

Red Kidney Beans—Dry, Cooked, Cooked without Fat ☛ Vitamin K = 15.1 mcg; DV= 12.6%; Serving size: 1 cup, 180 g

Red Kidney Beans—Dry, Cooked Made With Oil ☛ Vitamin K = 29 mcg; DV= 24.2%; Serving size: 1 cup, 180 g

Refried Beans—Made With Oil ☛ Vitamin K = 19.2 mcg; DV= 16%; Serving size: 1 cup, 253 g

Refried Beans—With Cheese ☛ Vitamin K = 5.3 mcg; DV= 4.4%; Serving size: 1 cup, 253 g

Refried Beans—With Meat ☛ Vitamin K = 6.1 mcg; DV= 5.1%; Serving size: 1 cup, 253 g

Soft Tofu ☛ Vitamin K = 2.4 mcg; DV= 2%; Serving size: 1 piece, 120 g

Soy—Flour Defatted ☛ Vitamin K = 4.3 mcg; DV= 3.6%; Serving size: 1 cup, 105 g

Soy—Flour Full-Fat Roasted ☛ Vitamin K = 60.4 mcg; DV= 50.3%; Serving size: 1 cup, stirred, 85 g

Soy—Flour Low-Fat ☛ Vitamin K = 3.4 mcg; DV= 2.8%; Serving size: 1 cup, stirred, 88 g

SoyBeans—Curd Breaded Fried ☛ Vitamin K = 1.5 mcg; DV= 1.3%; Serving size: 1 slice, 29 g

SoyBeans—Curd Cheese ☛ Vitamin K = 10.4 mcg; DV= 8.7%; Serving size: 1 cup, 225 g

Soybeans—Dry, Cooked, Cooked with Fat ☛ Vitamin K = 47.3 mcg; DV= 39.4%; Serving size: 1 cup, 180 g

Soybeans—Dry, Cooked, Cooked without Fat ☛ Vitamin K = 34.4 mcg; DV= 28.7%; Serving size: 1 cup, 180 g

Split Peas ☞ Vitamin K = 9.8 mcg; DV= 8.2%; Serving size: 1 cup, 196 g

Tofu Extra Firm Prepared With Nigari ☞ Vitamin K = 2.5 mcg; DV= 2.1%; Serving size: 1/5 block, 91 g

Tofu Fried ☞ Vitamin K = 2.2 mcg; DV= 1.8%; Serving size: 1 oz, 28.4 g

Tofu Yogurt ☞ Vitamin K = 9.2 mcg; DV= 7.7%; Serving size: 1 cup, 262 g

Vanilla Soy—Milk ☞ Vitamin K = 7.3 mcg; DV= 6.1%; Serving size: 1 cup, 243 g

Vegetarian Chili ☞ Vitamin K = 13 mcg; DV= 10.8%; Serving size: 1 cup, 254 g

Vegetarian Fillets ☞ Vitamin K = 0 mcg; DV= 0%; Serving size: 1 fillet, 85 g

Vegetarian Meatloaf Or Patties ☞ Vitamin K = 0 mcg; DV= 0%; Serving size: 1 slice, 56 g

Vegetarian Pot Pie ☞ Vitamin K = 26.1 mcg; DV= 21.8%; Serving size: 1 pie, 227 g

Vegetarian Stew ☞ Vitamin K = 41.2 mcg; DV= 34.3%; Serving size: 1 cup, 247 g

Vegetarian Stroganoff ☞ Vitamin K = 46.1 mcg; DV= 38.4%; Serving size: 1 box (3.2 oz), dry, yields, 466 g

Veggie Burgers ☞ Vitamin K = 2.9 mcg; DV= 2.4%; Serving size: 1 pattie, 70 g

Vermicelli Made From Soy ☞ Vitamin K = 5.3 mcg; DV= 4.4%; Serving size: 1 cup, 140 g

White Beans—Canned Drained, Cooked without Fat ☞ Vitamin K = 7.9 mcg; DV= 6.6%; Serving size: 1 cup, 180 g

White Beans—Canned Drained, Prepared With Oil or Margarine ☞ Vitamin K = 22.3 mcg; DV= 18.6%; Serving size: 1 cup, 180 g

White Beans—Dry, Cooked, Cooked without Fat ☞ Vitamin K = 6.3 mcg; DV= 5.3%; Serving size: 1 cup, 180 g

White Beans—Dry, Cooked Made With Oil ☞ Vitamin K = 20.7 mcg; DV= 17.3%; Serving size: 1 cup, 180 g

Yellow Canary Or Peruvian Beans—Dry, Cooked without Fat ☞ Vitamin K = 6.3 mcg; DV= 5.3%; Serving size: 1 cup, 180 g

Yellow Canary Or Peruvian Beans—Dry, Cooked Made With Oil ☞ Vitamin K = 20.7 mcg; DV= 17.3%; Serving size: 1 cup, 180 g

BEVERAGES

Abbott Eas Soy Protein Powder ☛ Vitamin K = 1.2 mcg; DV = 1%; Serving size: 1 scoop, 44 g

Abbott Eas Whey Protein Powder ☛ Vitamin K = 0.2 mcg; DV = 0.2%; Serving size: 2 scoop, 39 g

Abbott Ensure Nutritional Shake Ready-To-Drink ☛ Vitamin K = 21.3 mcg; DV = 17.8%; Serving size: 8 fl oz, 254 g

Abbott Ensure Plus Ready-To-Drink ☛ Vitamin K = 19.9 mcg; DV = 16.6%; Serving size: 1 cup, 252 g

Acai Berry Drink—Enriched ☛ Vitamin K = 44.4 mcg; DV = 37%; Serving size: 8 fl oz, 266 g

Alcoholic Beverage—Distilled All (Gin Rum Vodka Whiskey) 80 Proof ☛ Vitamin K = 0 mcg; DV = 0%; Serving size: 1 fl oz, 27.8 g

Alcoholic Beverage—Malt Beer ☛ Vitamin K = 0 mcg; DV = 0%; Serving size: fl oz, 335 g

Alcoholic Beverage—Wine ☛ Vitamin K = 0 mcg; DV = 0%; Serving size: 1 tsp, 4.9 g

Black Tea, Brewed, or Ready To Drink ☞ Vitamin K = 0 mcg; DV = 0%; Serving size: 1 fl oz, 29.6 g

Bottled Water ☞ Vitamin K = 0 mcg; DV = 0%; Serving size: 1 fl oz, 29.6 g

Carbonated—Beverage Chocolate-Flavored Soda ☞ Vitamin K = 0 mcg; DV = 0%; Serving size: 1 fl oz, 31 g

Chocolate Syrup ☞ Vitamin K = 0.2 mcg; DV = 0.2%; Serving size: 1 serving 2 tbsp, 39 g

Coffee ☞ Vitamin K = 0 mcg; DV = 0%; Serving size: 1 fl oz, 29.6 g

Coffee—Cafe Mocha With Non-Dairy Milk ☞ Vitamin K = 0.4 mcg; DV = 0.3%; Serving size: 1 fl oz, 31 g

Coffee—Cappuccino With Non-Dairy Milk ☞ Vitamin K = 0.2 mcg; DV = 0.2%; Serving size: 1 fl oz, 30 g

Coffee—Latte With Non-Dairy Milk ☞ Vitamin K = 0.4 mcg; DV = 0.3%; Serving size: 1 fl oz, 30 g

Cranberry Juice Cocktail Bottled ☞ Vitamin K = 0.3 mcg; DV = 0.3%; Serving size: 1 fl oz, 31.6 g

Cranberry-Apple Juice Drink—Bottled ☞ Vitamin K = 0.2 mcg; DV = 0.2%; Serving size: 1 fl oz, 30.6 g

Fruit Flavored Drink—Containing Less Than 3% Fruit Juice ☞ Vitamin K = 0 mcg; DV = 0%; Serving size: 1 cup (8 fl oz), 238 g

Fruit Juice Drink—Greater Than 3% Fruit Juice ☞ Vitamin K = 0 mcg; DV = 0%; Serving size: 8 fl oz, 237 g

Fruit Juice Drink—Noncitrus Carbonated ☞ Vitamin K = 0.4 mcg; DV = 0.3%; Serving size: 1 fl oz (no ice), 31 g

Fruit Smoothies—With Whole Fruit And Dairy ☞ Vitamin K = 0.9 mcg; DV = 0.8%; Serving size: 1 fl oz, 27 g

Fruit Smoothies—With Whole Fruit No Dairy ☛ Vitamin K = 1.2 mcg; DV = 1%; Serving size: 1 fl oz, 27 g

Lemonade—Flavor Drink—Powder ☛ Vitamin K = 0.3 mcg; DV = 0.3%; Serving size: 1 serving, 18 g

Milk And Soy Chocolate Drink ☛ Vitamin K = 40.1 mcg; DV = 33.4%; Serving size: 8 fl oz, 237 g

Nestle Boost Plus Nutritional Drink—Ready-To-Drink ☛ Vitamin K = 29.2 mcg; DV = 24.3%; Serving size: 1 bottle, 237 g

Nutritional Drink—High Protein Ready-To-Drink—(Slim Fast) ☛ Vitamin K = 16.1 mcg; DV = 13.4%; Serving size: 1 cup, 248 g

Nutritional Drink—High Protein Ready-To-Drink—Nfs ☛ Vitamin K = 16.6 mcg; DV = 13.8%; Serving size: 1 cup, 256 g

Nutritional Drink—Ready-To-Drink—(Carnation Instant Breakfast) ☛ Vitamin K = 29.8 mcg; DV = 24.8%; Serving size: 1 cup, 248 g

Nutritional Drink—Ready-To-Drink—(Kellogg's Special K Protein) ☛ Vitamin K = 2 mcg; DV = 1.7%; Serving size: 1 fl oz, 32 g

Nutritional Shake Mix High Protein Powder ☛ Vitamin K = 12.5 mcg; DV = 10.4%; Serving size: 1 tbsp, 10 g

Oatmeal Beverage With Milk or Water ☛ Vitamin K = 0.5 mcg; DV = 0.4%; Serving size: 1 cup, 248 g

Orange And Apricot Juice Drink—Canned ☛ Vitamin K = 0 mcg; DV = 0%; Serving size: 1 fl oz, 31.2 g

Orange Juice Drink ☛ Vitamin K = 0 mcg; DV = 0%; Serving size: 1 cup, 249 g

Tap Water ☛ Vitamin K = 0 mcg; DV = 0%; Serving size: 1 fl oz, 29.6 g

Tea—Green Brewed Regular ☛ Vitamin K = 0 mcg; DV = 0%; Serving size: 1 cup, 245 g

Tea—Green Instant or Ready to Drink ☛ Vitamin K = 0 mcg; DV = 0%; Serving size: 2 tbsp, 4.5 g

Tea—Herb Brewed Chamomile ☛ Vitamin K = 0 mcg; DV = 0%; Serving size: 1 fl oz, 29.6 g

Tea—Herb Other Than Chamomile Brewed ☛ Vitamin K = 0 mcg; DV = 0%; Serving size: 1 fl oz, 29.6 g

Tea—Hibiscus Brewed ☛ Vitamin K = 0 mcg; DV = 0%; Serving size: 8 fl oz, 237 g

Tea—Hot Chai With Milk ☛ Vitamin K = 0 mcg; DV = 0%; Serving size: 1 fl oz, 30 g

Whey Protein Powder—Isolate ☛ Vitamin K = 40 mcg; DV = 33.3%; Serving size: 3 scoop, 86 g

BREAKFAST CEREALS

Alpen ☞ Vitamin K = 1.4 mcg; DV = 1.2% ; Serving size: 2/3 cup (1 nlea serving), 55 g

Corn Flakes ☞ Vitamin K = 0 mcg; DV = 0% ; Serving size: 1 cup, 25 g

Crispy Brown Rice ☞ Vitamin K = 0 mcg; DV = 0% ; Serving size: 1 cup, 32 g

Frosted Corn Flakes ☞ Vitamin K = 0.1 mcg; DV = 0.1% ; Serving size: 1 cup, 40 g

Frosted Rice ☞ Vitamin K = 0 mcg; DV = 0% ; Serving size: 1 cup, 45 g

Granola ☞ Vitamin K = 2 mcg; DV = 1.7% ; Serving size: 1 cup, 111 g

Muesli ☞ Vitamin K = 1.4 mcg; DV = 1.2% ; Serving size: 1 cup, 85 g

Oat ☞ Vitamin K = 0.6 mcg; DV = 0.5% ; Serving size: 1 cup, nfs, 33 g

Puffed Wheat Sweetened ☞ Vitamin K = 1.1 mcg; DV = 0.9% ; Serving size: 1 cup, 38 g

Rice Flakes ☞ Vitamin K = 0 mcg; DV = 0% ; Serving size: 1 cup, 27 g

Corn Grits ☛ Vitamin K = 0 mcg; DV = 0% ; Serving size: 1 cup, 257 g

Cornmeal, Mush, Cooked with Fat ☛ Vitamin K = 2.2 mcg; DV = 1.8% ; Serving size: 1 cup, cooked, 240 g

Cornmeal, Mush, Cooked without Fat ☛ Vitamin K = 0 mcg; DV = 0% ; Serving size: 1 cup, cooked, 240 g

Cornmeal, Puerto Rican Style ☛ Vitamin K = 0.5 mcg; DV = 0.4% ; Serving size: 1 cup, cooked, 240 g

Cream Of Rice Dry ☛ Vitamin K = 0 mcg; DV = 0% ; Serving size: 1/4 cup (1 nlea serving), 45 g

Cream Of Rye ☛ Vitamin K = 1.7 mcg; DV = 1.4% ; Serving size: 1 cup, cooked, 240 g

Cream Of Wheat ☛ Vitamin K = 0 mcg; DV = 0% ; Serving size: 1 cup, 237 g

Cream Of Wheat—Instant Dry ☛ Vitamin K = 0.1 mcg; DV = 0.1% ; Serving size: 1 tbsp, 11.5 g

Frosted Oat ☛ Vitamin K = 0.4 mcg; DV = 0.3% ; Serving size: 3/4 cup (1 nlea serving), 30 g

Granola Homemade ☛ Vitamin K = 6.5 mcg; DV = 5.4% ; Serving size: 1 cup, 122 g

Grits, Regular or Instant, Cooked without Fat ☛ Vitamin K = 0.5 mcg; DV = 0.4% ; Serving size: 1 cup, cooked, 240 g

Grits, Regular or Instant, Cooked with Fat ☛ Vitamin K = 5.3 mcg; DV = 4.4% ; Serving size: 1 cup, cooked, 240 g

Hominy, Cooked with Fat ☛ Vitamin K = 2.4 mcg; DV = 2% ; Serving size: 1 cup, 170 g

Hominy, Cooked without Fat ☛ Vitamin K = 0.3 mcg; DV = 0.3% ; Serving size: 1 cup, 165 g

Masa Harina Cooked ☛ Vitamin K = 0 mcg; DV = 0% ; Serving size: 1 cup, cooked, 240 g

Millet Puffed ☛ Vitamin K = 0.3 mcg; DV = 0.3% ; Serving size: 1 cup, 21 g

Oatmeal, Instant Plain, Cooked with Fat ☛ Vitamin K = 4.8 mcg; DV = 4% ; Serving size: 1 cup, cooked, 240 g

Oatmeal, Instant Fruit Flavored, Cooked with Fat ☛ Vitamin K = 4.1 mcg; DV = 3.4% ; Serving size: 1 cup, cooked, 240 g

Oatmeal, Instant Fruit Flavored, Cooked without Fat ☛ Vitamin K = 1 mcg; DV = 0.8% ; Serving size: 1 cup, cooked, 240 g

Oats, Instant, Plain Dry ☛ Vitamin K = 0.5 mcg; DV = 0.4% ; Serving size: 1 packet, 28 g

Oats, Instant, Plain, Made With Water ☛ Vitamin K = 0.9 mcg; DV = 0.8% ; Serving size: 1 cup, cooked, 234 g

Oats, Regular And Quick, Dry ☛ Vitamin K = 1.6 mcg; DV = 1.3% ; Serving size: 1 cup, 81 g

Rice Cream Of, Cooked with Fat ☛ Vitamin K = 2.2 mcg; DV = 1.8% ; Serving size: 1 cup, cooked, 240 g

Rice Cream Of, Cooked without Fat ☛ Vitamin K = 0 mcg; DV = 0% ; Serving size: 1 cup, cooked, 240 g

Rice Cream Of, Cooked With Milk ☛ Vitamin K = 2.6 mcg; DV = 2.2% ; Serving size: 1 cup, cooked, 240 g

Toasted Wheat Germ ☛ Vitamin K = 1.1 mcg; DV = 0.9% ; Serving size: 1 oz, 28.4 g

Wheat Cream Of Cooked, Puerto Rican Style ☛ Vitamin K = 0.5 mcg; DV = 0.4% ; Serving size: 1 cup, cooked, 245 g

Wheatena Dry ☛ Vitamin K = 0.9 mcg; DV = 0.8% ; Serving size: 1/3 cup (1 nlea serving), 40 g

Whole Wheat, Cooked with Fat ☛ Vitamin K = 3.1 mcg; DV = 2.6% ; Serving size: 1 cup, cooked, 240 g

Whole Wheat, Cooked without Fat ☛ Vitamin K = 0.7 mcg; DV = 0.6% ; Serving size: 1 cup, cooked, 240 g

Whole Wheat, Dry ☛ Vitamin K = 2.3 mcg; DV = 1.9% ; Serving size: 1 cup, 94 g

DAIRY AND EGG PRODUCTS

Buttermilk ☛ Vitamin K = 0.7 mcg; DV = 0.6%; Serving size: 1 cup, 245 g

Camambert ☛ Vitamin K = 0.6 mcg; DV = 0.5%; Serving size: 1 oz, 28.4 g

Cheese, American ☛ Vitamin K = 3.8 mcg; DV = 3.2%; Serving size: 1 cup, 113 g

Cheese, American Cheddar Imitation ☛ Vitamin K = 0.6 mcg; DV = 0.5%; Serving size: 1 slice, 21 g

Cheese, Blue ☛ Vitamin K = 0.7 mcg; DV = 0.6%; Serving size: 1 oz, 28.4 g

Cheese, Brick Cheese ☛ Vitamin K = 3.3 mcg; DV = 2.8%; Serving size: 1 cup, diced, 132 g

Cheese, Brie ☛ Vitamin K = 0.7 mcg; DV = 0.6%; Serving size: 1 oz, 28.4 g

Cheese, Cheddar ☛ Vitamin K = 3.2 mcg; DV = 2.7%; Serving size: 1 cup, diced, 132 g

Cheese, Cheddar, Non-Fat ☛ Vitamin K = 0.2 mcg; DV = 0.2%; Serving size: 1 serving, 28 g

Cheese, Colby ☛ Vitamin K = 3.6 mcg; DV = 3%; Serving size: 1 cup, diced, 132 g

Cheese, Colby Jack ☛ Vitamin K = 0.2 mcg; DV = 0.2%; Serving size: 1 cracker-size slice, 9 g

Cheese, Cottage Cheese, With Gelatin Dessert And Fruit ☛ Vitamin K = 2.2 mcg; DV = 1.8%; Serving size: 1 cup, 240 g

Cheese, Cottage With Vegetables ☛ Vitamin K = 12.4 mcg; DV = 10.3%; Serving size: 4 oz, 113 g

Cheese, Cottage, (Blended) ☛ Vitamin K = 0 mcg; DV = 0%; Serving size: 4 oz, 113 g

Cheese, Cream Cheese ☛ Vitamin K = 0.3 mcg; DV = 0.3%; Serving size: 1 tbsp, 14.5 g

Cheese, Feta ☛ Vitamin K = 2.7 mcg; DV = 2.3%; Serving size: 1 cup, crumbled, 150 g

Cheese, Fontina ☛ Vitamin K = 3.4 mcg; DV = 2.8%; Serving size: 1 cup, diced, 132 g

Cheese, Goat ☛ Vitamin K = 3.4 mcg; DV = 2.8%; Serving size: 1 cup, crumbled, 140 g

Cheese, Gouda Or Edam ☛ Vitamin K = 0.2 mcg; DV = 0.2%; Serving size: 1 cracker-size slice, 9 g

Cheese, Gruyere ☛ Vitamin K = 0.8 mcg; DV = 0.7%; Serving size: 1 oz, 28.4 g

Cheese, Hard Goat ☛ Vitamin K = 0.9 mcg; DV = 0.8%; Serving size: 1 oz, 28.4 g

Cheese, Limburger ☛ Vitamin K = 3.1 mcg; DV = 2.6%; Serving size: 1 cup, 134 g

Cheese, Cheddar ☞ Vitamin K = 3.6 mcg; DV = 3%; Serving size: 1 cup, diced, 132 g

Cheese, Mexican Blend Cheese ☞ Vitamin K = 0.7 mcg; DV = 0.6%; Serving size: 1/4 cup shredded, 28 g

Cheese, Monterey ☞ Vitamin K = 3.3 mcg; DV = 2.8%; Serving size: 1 cup, diced, 132 g

Cheese, Mozzarella ☞ Vitamin K = 2.6 mcg; DV = 2.2%; Serving size: 1 cup, shredded, 112 g

Cheese, Muenster ☞ Vitamin K = 3.3 mcg; DV = 2.8%; Serving size: 1 cup, diced, 132 g

Cheese, Neufchatel ☞ Vitamin K = 0.5 mcg; DV = 0.4%; Serving size: 1 oz, 28.4 g

Cheese, Parmesan ☞ Vitamin K = 1.7 mcg; DV = 1.4%; Serving size: 1 cup, 100 g

Cheese, Processed American Cheese ☞ Vitamin K = 1.1 mcg; DV = 0.9%; Serving size: 1 oz, 28.4 g

Cheese, Processed Pimento Cheese ☞ Vitamin K = 4.1 mcg; DV = 3.4%; Serving size: 1 cup, diced, 140 g

Cheese, Processed Swiss Cheese ☞ Vitamin K = 3.1 mcg; DV = 2.6%; Serving size: 1 cup, diced, 140 g

Cheese, Provolone ☞ Vitamin K = 2.9 mcg; DV = 2.4%; Serving size: 1 cup, diced, 132 g

Cheese, Ricotta ☞ Vitamin K = 1.4 mcg; DV = 1.2%; Serving size: 1/2 cup, 124 g

Cheese, Romano ☞ Vitamin K = 0.6 mcg; DV = 0.5%; Serving size: 1 oz, 28.4 g

Cheese, Swiss ☞ Vitamin K = 1.8 mcg; DV = 1.5%; Serving size: 1 cup, diced, 132 g

Chocolate Milk (average value) ☞ Vitamin K = 2 mcg; DV = 1.7%; Serving size: 1 cup, 248 g

Cream—Half And Half Cream ☞ Vitamin K = 0.4 mcg; DV = 0.3%; Serving size: 1 fl oz, 30.2 g

Cream—Heavy Whipping Cream ☞ Vitamin K = 3.8 mcg; DV = 3.2%; Serving size: 1 cup, whipped, 120 g

Cream—Imitation Sour Cream ☞ Vitamin K = 1.4 mcg; DV = 1.2%; Serving size: 1 oz, 28.4 g

Dehydrated Milk ☞ Vitamin K = 0.7 mcg; DV = 0.6%; Serving size: 1/4 cup, 32 g

Egg Benedict ☞ Vitamin K = 5.2 mcg; DV = 4.3%; Serving size: 1 medium egg, 149 g

Egg Deviled ☞ Vitamin K = 3.3 mcg; DV = 2.8%; Serving size: 1/2 small egg, 24 g

Egg Duck Whole Fresh Raw ☞ Vitamin K = 0.3 mcg; DV = 0.3%; Serving size: 1 egg, 70 g

Egg Goose Whole Fresh Raw ☞ Vitamin K = 0.6 mcg; DV = 0.5%; Serving size: 1 egg, 144 g

Egg Omelet Or Scrambled Egg—Prepared With Oil or Margarine ☞ Vitamin K = 3.2 mcg; DV = 2.7%; Serving size: 1 small egg, 46 g

Egg Omelet Or Scrambled Egg—Prepared Without Fat ☞ Vitamin K = 0.1 mcg; DV = 0.1%; Serving size: 1 small egg, 44 g

Egg Omelet Or Scrambled Egg—With Cheese, And Dark-Green Vegetables Cooked with Fat ☞ Vitamin K = 23.5 mcg; DV = 19.6%; Serving size: 1 small egg, 62 g

Egg Omelet Or Scrambled Egg—With Cheese, And Dark-Green Vegetables Cooked without Fat ☞ Vitamin K = 20.5 mcg; DV = 17.1%; Serving size: 1 small egg, 60 g

Egg White Cooked Cooked with Fat ☛ Vitamin K = 1.4 mcg; DV = 1.2%; Serving size: 1 small egg white, 24 g

Egg White Cooked Cooked without Fat ☛ Vitamin K = 0 mcg; DV = 0%; Serving size: 1 small egg white, 24 g

Egg Whole Fried With Oil and Margarine ☛ Vitamin K = 3.1 mcg; DV = 2.6%; Serving size: 1 small, 35 g

Egg Yolk , Cooked with Fat ☛ Vitamin K = 1.2 mcg; DV = 1%; Serving size: 1 small egg yolk, 13 g

Egg Yolk Dried ☛ Vitamin K = 1 mcg; DV = 0.8%; Serving size: 1 cup, sifted, 67 g

Egg Yolk, Cooked without Fat ☛ Vitamin K = 0.1 mcg; DV = 0.1%; Serving size: 1 small egg yolk, 13 g

Ghee (Clarified Butter) ☛ Vitamin K = 1.1 mcg; DV = 0.9%; Serving size: 1 tbsp, 12.8 g

Goat Milk ☛ Vitamin K = 0.1 mcg; DV = 0.1%; Serving size: 1 fl oz, 30.5 g

Huevos Rancheros ☛ Vitamin K = 5.7 mcg; DV = 4.8%; Serving size: 1 egg, ns as to size, 118 g

Ice Cream—Bar Cake Covered ☛ Vitamin K = 4.2 mcg; DV = 3.5%; Serving size: 1 bar, 59 g

Ice Cream—Bar Stick Or Nugget With Crunch Coating ☛ Vitamin K = 21.2 mcg; DV = 17.7%; Serving size: 26 pieces, 95 g

Instant Breakfast Powder, Chocolate ☛ Vitamin K = 6.7 mcg; DV = 5.6%; Serving size: 1 tbsp, 5.6 g

Milk, Almond, Unsweetened ☛ Vitamin K = 0 mcg; DV = 0%; Serving size: 1 cup, 244 g

Milk, ButterMilk, Dried ☛ Vitamin K = 0.1 mcg; DV = 0.1%; Serving size: 1/4 cup, 30 g

Milk, Dry Reconstituted Whole ☞ Vitamin K = 0.7 mcg; DV = 0.6%; Serving size: 1 cup, 244 g

Milk, Dry Whole ☞ Vitamin K = 2.8 mcg; DV = 2.3%; Serving size: 1 cup, 128 g

Milk, Fluid 1% Fat ☞ Vitamin K = 0.2 mcg; DV = 0.2%; Serving size: 1 cup, 244 g

Milk, Shake Home Recipe (average value) ☞ Vitamin K = 0.1 mcg; DV = 0.1%; Serving size: 1 fl oz, 28 g

Milk, Skim ☞ Vitamin K = 0 mcg; DV = 0%; Serving size: 1 cup, 245 g

Salted Butter ☞ Vitamin K = 0.4 mcg; DV = 0.3%; Serving size: 1 pat, 5 g

Shrimp-Egg Patty ☞ Vitamin K = 5.5 mcg; DV = 4.6%; Serving size: 1 patty (2" dia), 18 g

Squash Summer Souffle ☞ Vitamin K = 3.1 mcg; DV = 2.6%; Serving size: 1 cup, 136 g

Squash Winter Souffle ☞ Vitamin K = 5.2 mcg; DV = 4.3%; Serving size: 1 cup, 157 g

Tofu Frozen Dessert (average value) ☞ Vitamin K = 5.9 mcg; DV = 4.9%; Serving size: 1 cup, 164 g

Unsalted Butter ☞ Vitamin K = 0.4 mcg; DV = 0.3%; Serving size: 1 pat, 5 g

Yogurt, Chocolate Nonfat Milk ☞ Vitamin K = 0 mcg; DV = 0%; Serving size: 1 container (6 oz), 170 g

Yogurt, Coconut Milk ☞ Vitamin K = 0 mcg; DV = 0%; Serving size: 1 6 oz container, 170 g

Yogurt, Fruit Reduced Fat ☞ Vitamin K = 2 mcg; DV = 1.7%; Serving size: 1 container (6 oz), 170 g

Yogurt, Fruit Variety Nonfat ☞ Vitamin K = 1.9 mcg; DV = 1.6%; Serving size: 1 container (6 oz), 170 g

Yogurt, Greek Reduced Fat with Fruit ☞ Vitamin K = 0 mcg; DV = 0%; Serving size: 1 tube, 57 g

Yogurt, Liquid ☞ Vitamin K = 0.1 mcg; DV = 0.1%; Serving size: 1 bottle, 93 g

Yogurt, Whole Milk, Fruit ☞ Vitamin K = 0.2 mcg; DV = 0.2%; Serving size: 1 4 oz container, 113 g

FAST-FOOD ITEMS

Bacon And Cheese Sandwich—With Spread ☛ Vitamin K = 9.1 mcg; DV = 7.6%; Serving size: 1 sandwich, 121 g

Bacon And Egg Sandwich ☛ Vitamin K = 3.4 mcg; DV = 2.8%; Serving size: 1 sandwich, 177 g

Bacon Breaded Fried Chicken Fillet And Tomato Club With Lettuce And Spread ☛ Vitamin K = 33.1 mcg; DV = 27.6%; Serving size: 1 sandwich, 227 g

Bacon Sandwich—With Spread ☛ Vitamin K = 7.5 mcg; DV = 6.3%; Serving size: 1 sandwich, 91 g

Blintz Cheese-Filled ☛ Vitamin K = 3 mcg; DV = 2.5%; Serving size: 1 blintz, 70 g

Blintz Fruit-Filled ☛ Vitamin K = 3.2 mcg; DV = 2.7%; Serving size: 1 blintz, 70 g

Bologna And Cheese Sandwich—With Spread ☛ Vitamin K = 8.1 mcg; DV = 6.8%; Serving size: 1 sandwich, 111 g

Bologna Sandwich—With Spread ☛ Vitamin K = 7.1 mcg; DV = 5.9%; Serving size: 1 sandwich, 83 g

Breadstick, Made With Garlic And Parmesan Cheese ☛ Vitamin K = 9.1 mcg; DV = 7.6%; Serving size: 1 breadstick, 43 g

Breakfast Burrito—With Egg Cheese And Sausage ☛ Vitamin K = 4.8 mcg; DV = 4%; Serving size: 1 burrito, 109 g

Breakfast Pizza With Egg ☛ Vitamin K = 6.2 mcg; DV = 5.2%; Serving size: 1 piece, nfs, 144 g

Bruschetta ☛ Vitamin K = 5 mcg; DV = 4.2%; Serving size: 1 slice, 43 g

Buffalo Chicken Submarine Sandwich ☛ Vitamin K = 35.5 mcg; DV = 29.6%; Serving size: 1 submarine, 240 g

Buffalo Chicken Submarine Sandwich—With Cheese ☛ Vitamin K = 34.8 mcg; DV = 29%; Serving size: 1 submarine, 260 g

Burger King—Cheeseburger ☛ Vitamin K = 7.6 mcg; DV = 6.3%; Serving size: 1 item, 133 g

Burger King—Chicken Strips ☛ Vitamin K = 2.3 mcg; DV = 1.9%; Serving size: 1 strip, 36 g

Burger King—Croissanwich With Egg And Cheese ☛ Vitamin K = 10.5 mcg; DV = 8.8%; Serving size: 1 item, 110 g

Burger King—Croissanwich With Sausage And Cheese ☛ Vitamin K = 8.5 mcg; DV = 7.1%; Serving size: 1 item, 131 g

Burger King—Croissanwich With Sausage Egg And Cheese ☛ Vitamin K = 16.2 mcg; DV = 13.5%; Serving size: 1 sandwich, 171 g

Burger King—Double Whopper No Cheese ☛ Vitamin K = 52.7 mcg; DV = 43.9%; Serving size: 1 item, 374 g

Burger King—Double Whopper With Cheese ☛ Vitamin K = 45.9 mcg; DV = 38.3%; Serving size: 1 item, 399 g

Burger King—French Fries ☛ Vitamin K = 8.2 mcg; DV = 6.8%; Serving size: 1 small serving, 74 g

Burger King—French Toast—Sticks ☛ Vitamin K = 3 mcg; DV = 2.5%; Serving size: 1 stick, 21 g

Burger King—Hamburger ☛ Vitamin K = 5.4 mcg; DV = 4.5%; Serving size: 1 sandwich, 99 g

Burger King—Original Chicken Sandwich ☛ Vitamin K = 47.2 mcg; DV = 39.3%; Serving size: 1 sandwich, 199 g

Burger King—Premium Fish Sandwich ☛ Vitamin K = 49.5 mcg; DV = 41.3%; Serving size: 1 sandwich, 220 g

Burger King—Whopper No Cheese ☛ Vitamin K = 56.7 mcg; DV = 47.3%; Serving size: 1 item, 291 g

Burger King—Whopper With Cheese ☛ Vitamin K = 60.4 mcg; DV = 50.3%; Serving size: 1 item, 316 g

Burrito—Taco Or Quesadilla (average value) ☛ Vitamin K = 7.2 mcg; DV = 6%; Serving size: 1 small, 110 g

Cheese Pizza ☛ Vitamin K = 7.2 mcg; DV = 6%; Serving size: 1 slice, 107 g

Cheeseburger (average value) ☛ Vitamin K = 18.9 mcg; DV = 15.8%; Serving size: 1 cheeseburger, 225 g

Chicken Breaded And Fried Boneless Pieces Plain ☛ Vitamin K = 6.7 mcg; DV = 5.6%; Serving size: 6 pieces, 96 g

Chicken Fillet Broiled Sandwich With Lettuce Tomato Spread ☛ Vitamin K = 18 mcg; DV = 15%; Serving size: 1 burger king sandwich, 155 g

Chicken Fillet Sandwich—Plain With Pickles ☛ Vitamin K = 15.9 mcg; DV = 13.3%; Serving size: 1 sandwich, 187 g

Chicken Patty Sandwich—Miniature With Spread ☞ Vitamin K = 5.4 mcg; DV = 4.5%; Serving size: 1 miniature sandwich, 31 g

Chicken Salad Or Chicken Spread Sandwich ☞ Vitamin K = 28.8 mcg; DV = 24%; Serving size: 1 sandwich, 141 g

Chicken Tenders ☞ Vitamin K = 2.4 mcg; DV = 2%; Serving size: 1 strip, 30 g

Coleslaw (Fast Food) ☞ Vitamin K = 135.4 mcg; DV = 112.8%; Serving size: 1 cup, 191 g

Corned Beef Sandwich ☞ Vitamin K = 13.8 mcg; DV = 11.5%; Serving size: 1 sandwich, 130 g

Crab Cake Sandwich—On Bun ☞ Vitamin K = 22.8 mcg; DV = 19%; Serving size: 1 sandwich, 140 g

Crispy Chicken In Tortilla With Lettuce Cheese ☞ Vitamin K = 31.4 mcg; DV = 26.2%; Serving size: 1 item, 133 g

Croissant Sandwich, Filled With Broccoli And Cheese ☞ Vitamin K = 16.4 mcg; DV = 13.7%; Serving size: 1 croissant, 113 g

Digiorno—Pizza Cheese (average value) ☞ Vitamin K = 13.8 mcg; DV = 11.5%; Serving size: 1 slice 1/4 of pie, 164 g

Domino's—14 Inch Cheese Pizza (average value) ☞ Vitamin K = 12.7 mcg; DV = 10.6%; Serving size: 1 slice, 108 g

Double Bacon Cheeseburger With condiments (average value) ☞ Vitamin K = 14.9 mcg; DV = 12.4%; Serving size: 1 double bacon cheeseburger, 275 g

Egg And Cheese On Biscuit ☞ Vitamin K = 11.8 mcg; DV = 9.8%; Serving size: 1 sandwich, 140 g

Egg And Steak On Biscuit ☞ Vitamin K = 12.7 mcg; DV = 10.6%; Serving size: 1 sandwich, 179 g

Egg Salad Sandwich ☛ Vitamin K = 51.4 mcg; DV = 42.8%; Serving size: 1 sandwich, 159 g

Fast Food—Pizza Chain 14 Inch Pizza (average value) ☛ Vitamin K = 10.9 mcg; DV = 9.1%; Serving size: 1 slice 1/8 pizza, 117 g

Fish Sandwich—With Tartar Sauce ☛ Vitamin K = 29.9 mcg; DV = 24.9%; Serving size: 1 sandwich, 220 g

Frankfurter Or Hot Dog Sandwich (average value) ☛ Vitamin K = 2.9 mcg; DV = 2.4%; Serving size: 1 frankfurter on bun, 102 g

French Toast (average value) ☛ Vitamin K = 3.8 mcg; DV = 3.2%; Serving size: 1 slice, any size, 65 g

Griddle Cake Sandwich (average value) ☛ Vitamin K = 3.5 mcg; DV = 2.9%; Serving size: 1 item 6.1 oz, 174 g

Grilled Chicken Bacon Club Sandwich, With Cheese Tomato and Lettuce ☛ Vitamin K = 23.3 mcg; DV = 19.4%; Serving size: 1 sandwich, 268 g

Grilled Chicken With Lettuce Cheese In Tortilla ☛ Vitamin K = 21.8 mcg; DV = 18.2%; Serving size: 1 item, 123 g

Gyro Sandwich ☛ Vitamin K = 14.8 mcg; DV = 12.3%; Serving size: 1 gyro, 390 g

Ham And Tomato Club Sandwich (With Lettuce) ☛ Vitamin K = 44.2 mcg; DV = 36.8%; Serving size: 1 sandwich, 254 g

Ham Salad Sandwich ☛ Vitamin K = 28.5 mcg; DV = 23.8%; Serving size: 1 sandwich, 141 g

Ham Sandwich—With Lettuce And Spread ☛ Vitamin K = 9.9 mcg; DV = 8.3%; Serving size: 1 sandwich, 127 g

Ham Sandwich—With Spread ☛ Vitamin K = 10.6 mcg; DV = 8.8%; Serving size: 1 sandwich, 112 g

Hamburger (average value) ☛ Vitamin K = 18 mcg; DV = 15%; Serving size: 1 hamburger, 200 g

KFC—Coleslaw ☛ Vitamin K = 79.4 mcg; DV = 66.2%; Serving size: 1 package, 112 g

KFC—Crispy Chicken Strips ☛ Vitamin K = 4.4 mcg; DV = 3.7%; Serving size: 1 strip, 47 g

KFC—Popcorn Chicken ☛ Vitamin K = 1.1 mcg; DV = 0.9%; Serving size: 1 piece, 6.4 g

Little Caesar's—14 Inch Cheese Pizza (average value) ☛ Vitamin K = 8 mcg; DV = 6.7%; Serving size: 1 slice, 102 g

McDonald's—Filet-O-Fish ☛ Vitamin K = 6.6 mcg; DV = 5.5%; Serving size: 1 sandwich, 134 g

McDonald's—French Fries ☛ Vitamin K = 11.4 mcg; DV = 9.5%; Serving size: 1 small serving, 71 g

Meat Sandwich (average value) ☛ Vitamin K = 7.1 mcg; DV = 5.9%; Serving size: 1 sandwich, 83 g

Nachos—With Cheese ☛ Vitamin K = 15.4 mcg; DV = 12.8%; Serving size: 1 serving, 80 g

Onion Rings Breaded And Fried ☛ Vitamin K = 65.3 mcg; DV = 54.4%; Serving size: 1 package (18 onion rings), 117 g

Pancakes (average value) ☛ Vitamin K = 1 mcg; DV = 0.8%; Serving size: 1 miniature/bite size pancake, 10 g

Papa John's—14 Inch Cheese Pizza (average value) ☛ Vitamin K = 8.8 mcg; DV = 7.3%; Serving size: 1 slice, 117 g

Pastrami Sandwich ☛ Vitamin K = 13.7 mcg; DV = 11.4%; Serving size: 1 sandwich, 134 g

Pepperoni And Salami Submarine Sandwich (With Lettuce) ☛ Vitamin K = 44.2 mcg; DV = 36.8%; Serving size: 1 submarine, 240 g

Pizza Hut—12 Inch Cheese Pizza (average value) ☞ Vitamin K = 11.6 mcg; DV = 9.7%; Serving size: 1 slice, 96 g

Pizza Hut—Breadstick—Parmesan Garlic ☞ Vitamin K = 9.1 mcg; DV = 7.6%; Serving size: 1 breadstick, 43 g

Potato—French Fries From Fresh Baked ☞ Vitamin K = 8.3 mcg; DV = 6.9%; Serving size: 1 serving small, 71 g

Potato—French Fries From Fresh Fried ☞ Vitamin K = 11.6 mcg; DV = 9.7%; Serving size: 1 serving small, 71 g

Potato—French Fries From Frozen Fried ☞ Vitamin K = 12.4 mcg; DV = 10.3%; Serving size: 1 serving small, 71 g

Potato—Hash Brown From Dry Mix ☞ Vitamin K = 28.6 mcg; DV = 23.8%; Serving size: 1 cup, 160 g

Potato—Hash Brown (average value) ☞ Vitamin K = 9.8 mcg; DV = 8.2%; Serving size: 1 patty, 55 g

Potato—Home Fries (average value) ☞ Vitamin K = 32.4 mcg; DV = 27%; Serving size: 1 cup, 200 g

Potato—Mashed ☞ Vitamin K = 14.3 mcg; DV = 11.9%; Serving size: 1 cup, 242 g

Potato—Patty ☞ Vitamin K = 5 mcg; DV = 4.2%; Serving size: 1 patty, 55 g

Potato—Skins (average value) ☞ Vitamin K = 2.1 mcg; DV = 1.8%; Serving size: skin from 1 small, 25 g

Potato—Tots (average value) ☞ Vitamin K = 13.8 mcg; DV = 11.5%; Serving size: 1 cup, 130 g

Puerto Rican Sandwich ☞ Vitamin K = 21.4 mcg; DV = 17.8%; Serving size: 1 sandwich, 160 g

Quesadilla With Chicken ☞ Vitamin K = 4.3 mcg; DV = 3.6%; Serving size: 1 each quesadilla, 180 g

Roast Beef Sandwich (average value) ☞ Vitamin K = 4.2 mcg; DV = 3.5%; Serving size: 1 sandwich, 149 g

Roast Beef Submarine Sandwich—With Cheese and Lettuce ☞ Vitamin K = 30.2 mcg; DV = 25.2%; Serving size: 1 submarine, 260 g

Roast Beef Submarine Sandwich—With Lettuce and Tomato ☞ Vitamin K = 28.8 mcg; DV = 24%; Serving size: 1 submarine, 240 g

Salami Sandwich With Spread ☞ Vitamin K = 7.9 mcg; DV = 6.6%; Serving size: 1 sandwich, 82 g

Sardine Sandwich—With Lettuce And Spread ☞ Vitamin K = 44.1 mcg; DV = 36.8%; Serving size: 1 sandwich, 214 g

Sausage Pizza ☞ Vitamin K = 7.8 mcg; DV = 6.5%; Serving size: 1 slice, 116 g

Sausage Sandwich ☞ Vitamin K = 0.1 mcg; DV = 0.1%; Serving size: 1 sandwich, 107 g

Shrimp Breaded And Fried ☞ Vitamin K = 1.8 mcg; DV = 1.5%; Serving size: 3 pieces shrimp, 39 g

Steak And Cheese Sandwich (average value), Without Lettuce ☞ Vitamin K = 6.5 mcg; DV = 5.4%; Serving size: 1 sandwich, 170 g

Steak Submarine Sandwich—With Lettuce And Tomato ☞ Vitamin K = 9.5 mcg; DV = 7.9%; Serving size: 1 sandwich, 186 g

Submarine Sandwich—Tuna On White Bread With Lettuce And Tomato ☞ Vitamin K = 53.1 mcg; DV = 44.3%; Serving size: 6-inch sub, 237 g

Submarine Sandwich—Turkey Breast With Lettuce And Tomato ☞ Vitamin K = 8.6 mcg; DV = 7.2%; Serving size: 6-inch sub, 184 g

Submarine Sandwich—Turkey Roast Beef And Ham With Lettuce And Tomato ☞ Vitamin K = 19.4 mcg; DV = 16.2%; Serving size: 12-inch sub, 413 g

Taco Bell—Bean Burrito ☛ Vitamin K = 7.8 mcg; DV = 6.5%; Serving size: 1 each burrito, 185 g

Taco Bell—Burrito (average value) ☛ Vitamin K = 14 mcg; DV = 11.7%; Serving size: 1 burrito, 241 g

Taco Bell—Nachos (average value) ☛ Vitamin K = 6 mcg; DV = 5%; Serving size: 1 serving, 80 g

Taco Bell—Original Taco (Beef Cheese And Lettuce) ☛ Vitamin K = 10.6 mcg; DV = 8.8%; Serving size: 1 each taco, 69 g

Taco Bell—Soft Taco (Beef Cheese And Lettuce) ☛ Vitamin K = 11.4 mcg; DV = 9.5%; Serving size: 1 each taco, 102 g

Taco Bell—Soft Taco (Chicken Cheese And Lettuce) ☛ Vitamin K = 8.5 mcg; DV = 7.1%; Serving size: 1 each taco, 98 g

Taco Bell—Soft Taco With Steak ☛ Vitamin K = 26.4 mcg; DV = 22%; Serving size: 1 item, 127 g

Taco Bell—Taco Salad ☛ Vitamin K = 57 mcg; DV = 47.5%; Serving size: 1 item, 533 g

Taco (Beef Cheese And Lettuce) ☛ Vitamin K = 10.6 mcg; DV = 8.8%; Serving size: 1 each taco, 69 g

Taquito Or Flauta With Egg ☛ Vitamin K = 2 mcg; DV = 1.7%; Serving size: 1 small taquito, 36 g

Tomato Sandwich ☛ Vitamin K = 21.8 mcg; DV = 18.2%; Serving size: 1 sandwich, 134 g

Tuna Melt Sandwich ☛ Vitamin K = 43.8 mcg; DV = 36.5%; Serving size: 1 sandwich, 150 g

Tuna Salad Sandwich (With Lettuce) ☛ Vitamin K = 23.4 mcg; DV = 19.5%; Serving size: 1 sandwich, 167 g

Turkey And Bacon Submarine Sandwich (average value) ☛ Vitamin K = 36.9 mcg; DV = 30.8%; Serving size: 1 submarine, 260 g

Turkey Or Chicken Burger With Condiments (average value) ☛ Vitamin K = 16.4 mcg; DV = 13.7%; Serving size: 1 sandwich, 200 g

Turkey Salad Or Turkey Spread Sandwich ☛ Vitamin K = 28.3 mcg; DV = 23.6%; Serving size: 1 sandwich, 141 g

Vegetable Submarine Sandwich, With Spread ☛ Vitamin K = 45.3 mcg; DV = 37.8%; Serving size: 1 submarine, 167 g

Waffle—Chocolate (average value) ☛ Vitamin K = 16.2 mcg; DV = 13.5%; Serving size: 2 waffles, 70 g

Waffle—Cinnamon ☛ Vitamin K = 11.8 mcg; DV = 9.8%; Serving size: 2 waffles, 70 g

Waffle—Fruit (average value) ☛ Vitamin K = 17.9 mcg; DV = 14.9%; Serving size: 2 waffles, 70 g

Waffle—Plain ☛ Vitamin K = 11.8 mcg; DV = 9.8%; Serving size: 2 waffles, 70 g

Waffle—Plain From Fast Food / Restaurant ☛ Vitamin K = 18.2 mcg; DV = 15.2%; Serving size: 2 waffles, 70 g

Waffle—Whole Grain ☛ Vitamin K = 12.3 mcg; DV = 10.3%; Serving size: 2 waffles, 70 g

Waffle—Whole Grain From Fast Food / Restaurant ☛ Vitamin K = 18.9 mcg; DV = 15.8%; Serving size: 2 waffles, 70 g

Waffle—Whole Grain From Frozen ☛ Vitamin K = 0.9 mcg; DV = 0.8%; Serving size: 1 miniature/bite size waffle, 10 g

Wendys—Chicken Nuggets ☛ Vitamin K = 5.4 mcg; DV = 4.5%; Serving size: 5 pieces, 68 g

Wendys—Classic Double With Cheese ☛ Vitamin K = 21.4 mcg; DV = 17.8%; Serving size: 1 item, 310 g

Wendys—Classic Single Hamburger No Cheese ☛ Vitamin K = 19.6 mcg; DV = 16.3%; Serving size: 1 item, 218 g

Wendys—Classic Single Hamburger With Cheese ☛ Vitamin K = 21.9 mcg; DV = 18.3%; Serving size: 1 item, 236 g

Wendys—French Fries ☛ Vitamin K = 4.5 mcg; DV = 3.8%; Serving size: 1 kid's meal serving, 71 g

Wendys—Frosty Dairy Dessert ☛ Vitamin K = 0.5 mcg; DV = 0.4%; Serving size: 1 junior 6 oz. cup, 113 g

Wendys—Homestyle Chicken Fillet Sandwich ☛ Vitamin K = 24.6 mcg; DV = 20.5%; Serving size: 1 item, 230 g

Wendys—Ultimate Chicken Grill Sandwich ☛ Vitamin K = 20 mcg; DV = 16.7%; Serving size: 1 item, 225 g

Wrap Sandwich—Filled With Beef Patty Cheese ☛ Vitamin K = 12.7 mcg; DV = 10.6%; Serving size: 1 snack wrap sandwich, 126 g

Wrap Sandwich—With Meat Poultry Or Fish Filled And Vegetables ☛ Vitamin K = 17.5 mcg; DV = 14.6%; Serving size: 1 sandwich, 240 g

Wrap Sandwich—With Meat Poultry Or Fish Filled Vegetables And Cheese ☛ Vitamin K = 18.8 mcg; DV = 15.7%; Serving size: 1 sandwich, 280 g

Wrap Sandwich—With Meat Poultry Or Fish Filled Vegetables And Rice ☛ Vitamin K = 74.5 mcg; DV = 62.1%; Serving size: 1 sandwich, 433 g

FATS AND OILS

Animal Fat Or Drippings ☛ Vitamin K = 1.2 mcg; DV =1%; Serving size: 1 cup, 205 g

Bacon Grease ☛ Vitamin K = 0 mcg; DV =0%; Serving size: 1 tsp, 4.3 g

Beef Tallow ☛ Vitamin K = 0 mcg; DV =0%; Serving size: 1 tbsp, 12.8 g

Butter Light Stick ☛ Vitamin K = 0.7 mcg; DV =0.6%; Serving size: 1 tablespoon, 14 g

Butter-Margarine—Blend Stick Salted or unsalted ☛ Vitamin K = 113.5 mcg; DV =94.6%; Serving size: 1 cup, 227 g

Cocoa Butter ☛ Vitamin K = 3.4 mcg; DV =2.8%; Serving size: 1 tablespoon, 13.6 g

Creamy Poppyseed Salad Dressing ☛ Vitamin K = 16.6 mcg; DV =13.8%; Serving size: 2 tbsp, 33 g

Lard ☛ Vitamin K = 0 mcg; DV =0%; Serving size: 1 tbsp, 12.8 g

Margarine-Like Blend Soybean Oil And Butter ☞ Vitamin K = 12.2 mcg; DV =10.2%; Serving size: 1 tbsp, 14.1 g

Margarine-Like Shortening ☞ Vitamin K = 6 mcg; DV =5%; Serving size: 1 tbsp, 14 g

Margarine-Like Spread (average value) ☞ Vitamin K = 12.4 mcg; DV =10.3%; Serving size: 1 tbsp, 14 g

Margarine-Like Vegetable Oil-Butter Spread (average value) ☞ Vitamin K = 14.1 mcg; DV =11.8%; Serving size: 1 tbsp, 14 g

Margarine—(Unsalted) ☞ Vitamin K = 13.2 mcg; DV =11%; Serving size: 1 tbsp, 14.2 g

Margarine—Partially Hydrogenated For Flaky Pastries ☞ Vitamin K = 14.9 mcg; DV =12.4%; Serving size: 1 tbsp, 14 g

Mayonnaise Reduced-Fat Made With Olive Oil ☞ Vitamin K = 8.1 mcg; DV =6.8%; Serving size: 1 tbsp, 15 g

Mayonnaise Reduced Calorie ☞ Vitamin K = 3.5 mcg; DV =2.9%; Serving size: 1 tbsp, 14 g

Mayonnaise Prepared With Tofu ☞ Vitamin K = 8 mcg; DV =6.7%; Serving size: 1 tbsp, 15 g

Oil—Almond ☞ Vitamin K = 1 mcg; DV =0.8%; Serving size: 1 tablespoon, 13.6 g

Oil—Canola ☞ Vitamin K = 10 mcg; DV =8.3%; Serving size: 1 tbsp, 14 g

Oil—Coconut ☞ Vitamin K = 0.1 mcg; DV =0.1%; Serving size: 1 tbsp, 13.6 g

Oil—Corn ☞ Vitamin K = 0.3 mcg; DV =0.3%; Serving size: 1 tbsp, 13.6 g

Oil—Corn And Canola ☞ Vitamin K = 5.9 mcg; DV =4.9%; Serving size: 1 tbsp, 14 g

Oil—Corn Peanut And Olive ☛ Vitamin K = 2.9 mcg; DV =2.4%; Serving size: 1 tablespoon, 14 g

Oil—Cottonseed ☛ Vitamin K = 3.4 mcg; DV =2.8%; Serving size: 1 tablespoon, 13.6 g

Oil—Flaxseed ☛ Vitamin K = 1.3 mcg; DV =1.1%; Serving size: 1 tbsp, 13.6 g

Oil—Oat ☛ Vitamin K = 3.4 mcg; DV =2.8%; Serving size: 1 tbsp, 13.6 g

Oil—Olive ☛ Vitamin K = 8.1 mcg; DV =6.8%; Serving size: 1 tablespoon, 13.5 g

Oil—Palm ☛ Vitamin K = 1.1 mcg; DV =0.9%; Serving size: 1 tbsp, 13.6 g

Oil—Palm Kernel ☛ Vitamin K = 3.4 mcg; DV =2.8%; Serving size: 1 tablespoon, 13.6 g

Oil—Peanut ☛ Vitamin K = 0.1 mcg; DV =0.1%; Serving size: 1 tbsp, 13.5 g

Oil—Rice Bran ☛ Vitamin K = 3.4 mcg; DV =2.8%; Serving size: 1 tablespoon, 13.6 g

Oil—Safflower ☛ Vitamin K = 1 mcg; DV =0.8%; Serving size: 1 tablespoon, 13.6 g

Oil—Sesame ☛ Vitamin K = 1.8 mcg; DV =1.5%; Serving size: 1 tablespoon, 13.6 g

Oil—Soybean ☛ Vitamin K = 25 mcg; DV =20.8%; Serving size: 1 tbsp, 13.6 g

Oil—Sunflower Linoleic (average value) ☛ Vitamin K = 0.7 mcg; DV =0.6%; Serving size: 1 tbsp, 13.6 g

Oil—Walnut ☛ Vitamin K = 2 mcg; DV =1.7%; Serving size: 1 tbsp, 13.6 g

Oil—Wheat Germ ☞ Vitamin K = 1.1 mcg; DV =0.9%; Serving size: 1 tsp, 4.5 g

Mayonnaise ☞ Vitamin K = 6.2 mcg; DV =5.2%; Serving size: 1 tbsp, 14.7 g

Table Fat (average value) ☞ Vitamin K = 101.5 mcg; DV =84.6%; Serving size: 1 cup, 227 g

Tartar Sauce Reduced-Fat/calorie ☞ Vitamin K = 64.3 mcg; DV =53.6%; Serving size: 1 cup, 224 g

Thousand Island ☞ Vitamin K = 11.1 mcg; DV =9.3%; Serving size: 1 tbsp, 16 g

Vegetable Oil-Butter Spread Reduced Calorie ☞ Vitamin K = 7.9 mcg; DV =6.6%; Serving size: 1 tbsp, 13 g

Vegetable Oil-Butter Spread Stick Salted ☞ Vitamin K = 223.6 mcg; DV =186.3%; Serving size: 1 cup, 227 g

Vegetable Shortening ☞ Vitamin K = 6.8 mcg; DV =5.7%; Serving size: 1 tbsp, 12.8 g

FINFISH AND SHELLFISH PRODUCTS

Anchovies, Canned In Oil ☛ Vitamin K = 64.2 mcg; DV = 53.5%; Serving size: 1 cup, solid or chunks, 146 g

Anchovies Raw ☛ Vitamin K = 0.1 mcg; DV = 0.1%; Serving size: 3 oz, 85 g

Barracuda, Coated Fried (With Oil or Margarine) ☛ Vitamin K = 12.9 mcg; DV = 10.8%; Serving size: 1 small fillet, 113 g

Barracuda, Coated without Fat (average value) ☛ Vitamin K = 0.9 mcg; DV = 0.8%; Serving size: 1 small fillet, 113 g

Barracuda, Cooked with Fat (average value) ☛ Vitamin K = 8.2 mcg; DV = 6.8%; Serving size: 1 small fillet, 113 g

Bouillabaisse ☛ Vitamin K = 21.3 mcg; DV = 17.8%; Serving size: 1 cup, 227 g

Carp, Coated Fried (With Oil or Margarine) ☛ Vitamin K = 19.4 mcg; DV = 16.2%; Serving size: 1 small fillet, 170 g

Carp, Cooked with Fat (average value) ☛ Vitamin K = 12.4 mcg; DV = 10.3%; Serving size: 1 small fillet, 170 g

Carp, Cooked Without Fat ☞ Vitamin K = 0.6 mcg; DV = 0.5%; Serving size: 3 oz, 85 g

Catfish Channel Farmed Raw ☞ Vitamin K = 1.8 mcg; DV = 1.5%; Serving size: 3 oz, 85 g

Catfish, Coated Fried (With Oil or Margarine) ☞ Vitamin K = 14.8 mcg; DV = 12.3%; Serving size: 1 small fillet, 113 g

Catfish, Cooked with Fat (average value) ☞ Vitamin K = 8.8 mcg; DV = 7.3%; Serving size: 1 small fillet, 113 g

Caviar Black And Red Granular ☞ Vitamin K = 0.1 mcg; DV = 0.1%; Serving size: 1 tbsp, 16 g

Ceviche ☞ Vitamin K = 10.3 mcg; DV = 8.6%; Serving size: 1 cup, 250 g

Cisco Smoked ☞ Vitamin K = 0 mcg; DV = 0%; Serving size: 1 oz, 28.4 g

Clam Cake Or Patty ☞ Vitamin K = 28.8 mcg; DV = 24%; Serving size: 1 cake or patty, 120 g

Clams, Coated Fried (With Oil or Margarine) ☞ Vitamin K = 3.3 mcg; DV = 2.8%; Serving size: 1 oz (without shell, cooked), 28 g

Clams, Coated, Cooked without Fat) ☞ Vitamin K = 0.2 mcg; DV = 0.2%; Serving size: 1 oz (without shell, cooked), 28 g

Clams, Cooked with Fat (average value) ☞ Vitamin K = 2 mcg; DV = 1.7%; Serving size: 1 oz (without shell, cooked), 28 g

Clams, Cooked without Fat ☞ Vitamin K = 0.1 mcg; DV = 0.1%; Serving size: 1 oz (without shell, cooked), 28 g

Cod, Coated Fried (without Fat) ☞ Vitamin K = 2 mcg; DV = 1.7%; Serving size: 1 small fillet, 170 g

Cod, Coated Fried (With Oil or Margarine) ☞ Vitamin K = 19.2 mcg; DV = 16%; Serving size: 1 small fillet, 170 g

Cod, Cooked with Fat (average value) ☛ Vitamin K = 13.1 mcg; DV = 10.9%; Serving size: 1 small fillet, 170 g

Codfish Ball Or Cake ☛ Vitamin K = 5.1 mcg; DV = 4.3%; Serving size: 1 ball, 63 g

Codfish Salad Puerto Rican Style Serenata ☛ Vitamin K = 16.7 mcg; DV = 13.9%; Serving size: 1 cup, 145 g

Codfish With Starchy Vegetables ☛ Vitamin K = 8 mcg; DV = 6.7%; Serving size: 1 cup, 173 g

Crab Deviled ☛ Vitamin K = 41 mcg; DV = 34.2%; Serving size: 1 cup, 175 g

Crab Imperial ☛ Vitamin K = 15.5 mcg; DV = 12.9%; Serving size: 1 cup, 259 g

Crab Salad ☛ Vitamin K = 84 mcg; DV = 70%; Serving size: 1 cup, 208 g

Crab Soft Shell, Coated Fried (With Oil or Margarine) ☛ Vitamin K = 3.4 mcg; DV = 2.8%; Serving size: 1 oz, cooked, 28 g

Crab, Cooked with Fat (average value) ☛ Vitamin K = 9 mcg; DV = 7.5%; Serving size: 1 cup (cooked, flaked and pieces), 118 g

Crayfish, Coated Fried (With Oil or Margarine) ☛ Vitamin K = 3.3 mcg; DV = 2.8%; Serving size: 1 oz (without shell, cooked), 28 g

Croaker Atlantic Raw ☛ Vitamin K = 0.1 mcg; DV = 0.1%; Serving size: 1 fillet, 79 g

Croaker, Coated Fried (With Oil or Margarine) ☛ Vitamin K = 12.9 mcg; DV = 10.8%; Serving size: 1 small fillet, 113 g

Croaker, Cooked with Fat (average value) ☛ Vitamin K = 8.2 mcg; DV = 6.8%; Serving size: 1 small fillet, 113 g

Croaker, Cooked without Fat ☛ Vitamin K = 0.8 mcg; DV = 0.7%; Serving size: 1 small fillet, 113 g

Eel Mixed Species Raw ☛ Vitamin K = 0 mcg; DV = 0%; Serving size: 3 oz, 85 g

Eel Smoked ☛ Vitamin K = 0 mcg; DV = 0%; Serving size: 1 oz, boneless, 28 g

Eel, Cooked without Fat (average value) ☛ Vitamin K = 0.3 mcg; DV = 0.3%; Serving size: 1 oz, boneless, raw, 23 g

Farmed Atlantic Salmon (Raw) ☛ Vitamin K = 0.4 mcg; DV = 0.3%; Serving size: 3 oz, 85 g

Fish Raw, Steamed, Boiled or Poached ☛ Vitamin K = 0.3 mcg; DV = 0.3%; Serving size: 1 small fillet, 113 g

Fish Curry ☛ Vitamin K = 115.9 mcg; DV = 96.6%; Serving size: 1 cup, 236 g

Fish Tofu And Vegetables Tempura ☛ Vitamin K = 18.6 mcg; DV = 15.5%; Serving size: 1 cup, 63 g

Flat Fish (Flounder Or Sole), , Cooked without Fat (average value) ☛ Vitamin K = 1.9 mcg; DV = 1.6%; Serving size: 1 fillet, 127 g

Flounder With Chopped Broccoli Diet Frozen Meal ☛ Vitamin K = 119 mcg; DV = 99.2%; Serving size: 1 meal (12.4 oz), 351 g

Flounder With Crab Stuffing ☛ Vitamin K = 30.5 mcg; DV = 25.4%; Serving size: 1 piece, 210 g

Flounder, Coated Fried (average value) ☛ Vitamin K = 12.9 mcg; DV = 10.8%; Serving size: 1 small fillet, 113 g

Flounder, Cooked with Fat (average value) ☛ Vitamin K = 8.2 mcg; DV = 6.8%; Serving size: 1 small fillet, 113 g

Flounder, Cooked without Fat (average value) ☛ Vitamin K = 1.2 mcg; DV = 1%; Serving size: 1 small fillet, 113 g

Fried Fish With Sauce Puerto Rican Style ☛ Vitamin K = 12.4 mcg; DV = 10.3%; Serving size: 1 slice, 213 g

Frog Legs Raw ☛ Vitamin K = 0 mcg; DV = 0%; Serving size: 1 leg, 45 g

Gefilte Fish ☛ Vitamin K = 0.5 mcg; DV = 0.4%; Serving size: 1 cup, 227 g

Gumbo (average value) ☛ Vitamin K = 12.9 mcg; DV = 10.8%; Serving size: 1 cup, 244 g

Haddock Cake Or Patty ☛ Vitamin K = 7.2 mcg; DV = 6%; Serving size: 1 cake or patty, 120 g

Haddock With Chopped Spinach Diet Frozen Meal ☛ Vitamin K = 104 mcg; DV = 86.7%; Serving size: 1 meal (9 oz), 255 g

Haddock, Coated Fried (With Oil or Margarine) ☛ Vitamin K = 19.4 mcg; DV = 16.2%; Serving size: 1 small fillet, 170 g

Haddock, Cooked without Fat (average value) ☛ Vitamin K = 1.9 mcg; DV = 1.6%; Serving size: 1 small fillet, 170 g

Halibut, Cooked with Fat (average value) ☛ Vitamin K = 12.2 mcg; DV = 10.2%; Serving size: 1 small fillet, 170 g

Halibut, Cooked without Fat (average value) ☛ Vitamin K = 2.2 mcg; DV = 1.8%; Serving size: 1 small fillet, 170 g

Herring Atlantic Raw ☛ Vitamin K = 0 mcg; DV = 0%; Serving size: 1 oz, boneless, 28.4 g

Herring, Cooked with Fat (average value) ☛ Vitamin K = 1.7 mcg; DV = 1.4%; Serving size: 1 oz, boneless, raw, 23 g

Herring, Cooked without Fat (average value) ☛ Vitamin K = 0.3 mcg; DV = 0.3%; Serving size: 1 oz, boneless, raw, 23 g

Lobster Gumbo ☛ Vitamin K = 21.7 mcg; DV = 18.1%; Serving size: 1 cup, 244 g

Lobster Newburg ☛ Vitamin K = 4.1 mcg; DV = 3.4%; Serving size: 1 cup, 244 g

Lobster Northern Raw ☛ Vitamin K = 0 mcg; DV = 0%; Serving size: 1 lobster, 150 g

Lobster Salad ☛ Vitamin K = 70.6 mcg; DV = 58.8%; Serving size: 1 cup, 182 g

Lobster, Cooked ☛ Vitamin K = 0 mcg; DV = 0%; Serving size: 1 cup, 145 g

Lomi Salmon ☛ Vitamin K = 54.1 mcg; DV = 45.1%; Serving size: 1 cup, 234 g

Mackerel Cake Or Patty ☛ Vitamin K = 7.9 mcg; DV = 6.6%; Serving size: 1 cake or patty, 120 g

Mackerel Raw ☛ Vitamin K = 1 mcg; DV = 0.8%; Serving size: 1 oz, boneless, raw, 28 g

Mackerel Salted ☛ Vitamin K = 6.2 mcg; DV = 5.2%; Serving size: 1 piece, 80 g

Mackerel, Pickled ☛ Vitamin K = 7.1 mcg; DV = 5.9%; Serving size: 3 oz, boneless, 84 g

Mackerel, Coated Fried (With Oil or Margarine) ☛ Vitamin K = 24 mcg; DV = 20%; Serving size: 1 small fillet, 170 g

Mackerel, Cooked with Fat (average value) ☛ Vitamin K = 12.6 mcg; DV = 10.5%; Serving size: 1 small fillet, 170 g

Mackerel, Cooked without Fat (average value) ☛ Vitamin K = 2 mcg; DV = 1.7%; Serving size: 1 small fillet, 170 g

Mollusks Abalone Floured Or Breaded Fried ☛ Vitamin K = 9 mcg; DV = 7.5%; Serving size: 1 oz, cooked, 28 g

Mollusks Abalone Mixed Species Raw ☛ Vitamin K = 19.6 mcg; DV = 16.3%; Serving size: 3 oz, 85 g

Mollusks Abalone, Steamed Or Poached ☛ Vitamin K = 12.8 mcg; DV = 10.7%; Serving size: 1 oz, cooked, 28 g

Mollusks Mussel Blue Raw ☞ Vitamin K = 0.2 mcg; DV = 0.2%; Serving size: 1 cup, 150 g

Mollusks Oyster Eastern Wild Raw ☞ Vitamin K = 0.8 mcg; DV = 0.7%; Serving size: 6 medium, 84 g

Mollusks Snail Raw ☞ Vitamin K = 0.1 mcg; DV = 0.1%; Serving size: 3 oz, 85 g

Mollusks Whelk Unspecified Raw ☞ Vitamin K = 0.1 mcg; DV = 0.1%; Serving size: 3 oz, 85 g

Mullet, Coated Fried (With Oil or Margarine) ☞ Vitamin K = 12.9 mcg; DV = 10.8%; Serving size: 1 small fillet, 113 g

Mullet, Cooked with Fat (average value) ☞ Vitamin K = 8.2 mcg; DV = 6.8%; Serving size: 1 small fillet, 113 g

Mullet, Cooked without Fat (average value) ☞ Vitamin K = 1.6 mcg; DV = 1.3%; Serving size: 1 small fillet, 113 g

Octopus Salad Puerto Rican Style ☞ Vitamin K = 17.6 mcg; DV = 14.7%; Serving size: 1 cup, 180 g

Octopus Smoked, Dried, Steamed, or Cooked without Fat (average value) ☞ Vitamin K = 0.7 mcg; DV = 0.6%; Serving size: 1 oz, boneless, cooked, 28 g

Octopus, Dried ☞ Vitamin K = 0.1 mcg; DV = 0.1%; Serving size: 1 oz, 28 g

Oyster Fritter ☞ Vitamin K = 9.7 mcg; DV = 8.1%; Serving size: 1 fritter, 40 g

Oysters Rockefeller ☞ Vitamin K = 37.7 mcg; DV = 31.4%; Serving size: 1 oyster, no shell, 24 g

Oysters Smoked, Or Steamed ☞ Vitamin K = 0.4 mcg; DV = 0.3%; Serving size: 1 oz, 28 g

Oysters, Coated Fried (With Oil or Margarine) ☞ Vitamin K = 3.5

mcg; DV = 2.9%; Serving size: 1 oz (without shell, cooked), 28 g

Oysters, Cooked with Fat (average value) ☛ Vitamin K = 2.1 mcg; DV = 1.8%; Serving size: 1 oz (without shell, cooked), 28 g

Oysters, Cooked without Fat (average value) ☛ Vitamin K = 0.3 mcg; DV = 0.3%; Serving size: 1 oz (without shell), 28 g

Perch All Species, Coated Fried (With Oil or Margarine) ☛ Vitamin K = 12.9 mcg; DV = 10.8%; Serving size: 1 small fillet, 113 g

Perch All Species, Cooked with Fat (average value) ☛ Vitamin K = 8.2 mcg; DV = 6.8%; Serving size: 1 small fillet, 113 g

Perch All Species, Cooked without Fat (average value) ☛ Vitamin K = 1.2 mcg; DV = 1%; Serving size: 1 small fillet, 113 g

Pike, Coated Fried (With Oil or Margarine) ☛ Vitamin K = 19.4 mcg; DV = 16.2%; Serving size: 1 small fillet, 170 g

Pike, Cooked with Fat (average value) ☛ Vitamin K = 12.4 mcg; DV = 10.3%; Serving size: 1 small fillet, 170 g

Pike, Cooked without Fat (average value) ☛ Vitamin K = 2.6 mcg; DV = 2.2%; Serving size: 1 small fillet, 170 g

Pollock Atlantic Raw ☛ Vitamin K = 0.1 mcg; DV = 0.1%; Serving size: 3 oz, 85 g

Pompano, Cooked with Fat (average value) ☛ Vitamin K = 2.5 mcg; DV = 2.1%; Serving size: 1 small fillet, 113 g

Pompano, Cooked with Fat (average value) ☛ Vitamin K = 8.2 mcg; DV = 6.8%; Serving size: 1 small fillet, 113 g

Porgy, Coated Fried (With Oil or Margarine) ☛ Vitamin K = 12.9 mcg; DV = 10.8%; Serving size: 1 small fillet, 113 g

Porgy, Cooked with Fat (average value) ☛ Vitamin K = 8.5 mcg; DV = 7.1%; Serving size: 1 small fillet, 113 g

Porgy, Cooked with Fat (average value) ☛ Vitamin K = 7.9 mcg; DV = 6.6%; Serving size: 1 small fillet, 113 g

Rainbow Trout (Raw) ☛ Vitamin K = 0.1 mcg; DV = 0.1%; Serving size: 1 fillet, 79 g

Ray, Coated Fried (With Oil or Margarine) ☛ Vitamin K = 3.1 mcg; DV = 2.6%; Serving size: 1 oz, boneless, raw, 27 g

Ray, Cooked with Fat (average value) ☛ Vitamin K = 1.8 mcg; DV = 1.5%; Serving size: 1 oz, boneless, raw, 23 g

Ray, Cooked with Fat (average value) ☛ Vitamin K = 1.6 mcg; DV = 1.3%; Serving size: 1 oz, boneless, raw, 23 g

Rockfish Pacific Mixed Species Raw ☛ Vitamin K = 0 mcg; DV = 0%; Serving size: 3 oz, 85 g

Roe ☛ Vitamin K = 0 mcg; DV = 0%; Serving size: 1 tbsp, 14 g

Roe, Cooked with Fat (average value) ☛ Vitamin K = 2.1 mcg; DV = 1.8%; Serving size: 1 oz, 28 g

Roughy Orange Raw ☛ Vitamin K = 0.6 mcg; DV = 0.5%; Serving size: 3 oz, 85 g

Salmon Cake Or Patty ☛ Vitamin K = 15.1 mcg; DV = 12.6%; Serving size: 1 ball, 63 g

Salmon Loaf ☛ Vitamin K = 18 mcg; DV = 15%; Serving size: 1 slice, 105 g

Salmon Salad ☛ Vitamin K = 89.4 mcg; DV = 74.5%; Serving size: 1 cup, 208 g

Salmon, Coated Fried (With Oil or Margarine), Prepared with Fat ☛ Vitamin K = 19.7 mcg; DV = 16.4%; Serving size: 1 small fillet, 170 g

Salmon, Coated Fried, Prepared without Fat ☛ Vitamin K = 2.7 mcg; DV = 2.3%; Serving size: 1 small fillet, 170 g

Salmon, Cooked with Fat (average value) ☛ Vitamin K = 13.3 mcg; DV = 11.1%; Serving size: 1 small fillet, 170 g

Salmon, Dried, Smoked, Steamed or Poached ☛ Vitamin K = 0.3 mcg; DV = 0.3%; Serving size: 1 oz, boneless, 28 g

Sardine All Species, Raw ☛ Vitamin K = 0.4 mcg; DV = 0.3%; Serving size: 1 cup, 89 g

Sardine, Canned In Oil ☛ Vitamin K = 64.2 mcg; DV = 53.5%; Serving size: 1 cup, solid or chunks, 146 g

Sardines, Dried ☛ Vitamin K = 0.1 mcg; DV = 0.1%; Serving size: 1 oz, 28 g

Scallops, Coated Fried (With Oil or Margarine) ☛ Vitamin K = 3.3 mcg; DV = 2.8%; Serving size: 1 oz, cooked, 28 g

Scallops, Cooked with Fat (average value) ☛ Vitamin K = 10.2 mcg; DV = 8.5%; Serving size: 1 cup, raw, yield cooked, 144 g

Scallops, Cooked without Fat (average value) ☛ Vitamin K = 6 mcg; DV = 5%; Serving size: 1 cup, 144 g

Scup Raw ☛ Vitamin K = 0.1 mcg; DV = 0.1%; Serving size: 3 oz, 85 g

Sea Bass, Coated Fried (With Oil or Margarine) ☛ Vitamin K = 12.9 mcg; DV = 10.8%; Serving size: 1 small fillet, 113 g

Sea Bass, Pickled ☛ Vitamin K = 1.6 mcg; DV = 1.3%; Serving size: 1 oz, boneless, 28 g

Sea Bass, Cooked with Fat (average value) ☛ Vitamin K = 8 mcg; DV = 6.7%; Serving size: 1 small fillet, 113 g

Sea Bass, Cooked without Fat (average value) ☛ Vitamin K = 5.1 mcg; DV = 4.3%; Serving size: 1 small fillet, 113 g

Seafood Garden Salad With Lettuce Tomato Carrots And Vegetables ☛ Vitamin K = 68.3 mcg; DV = 56.9%; Serving size: 1 cup, 95 g

Seafood Garden Salad With Lettuce Vegetables Without Tomato And

Carrots ☛ Vitamin K = 72.3 mcg; DV = 60.3%; Serving size: 1 cup, 95 g

Seafood Salad (average value) ☛ Vitamin K = 83.6 mcg; DV = 69.7%; Serving size: 1 cup, 208 g

Shark, Coated Fried (With Oil or Margarine) ☛ Vitamin K = 19.4 mcg; DV = 16.2%; Serving size: 1 small fillet, 170 g

Shark, Cooked with Fat (average value) ☛ Vitamin K = 12.4 mcg; DV = 10.3%; Serving size: 1 small fillet, 170 g

Shark, Cooked without Fat (average value) ☛ Vitamin K = 0.2 mcg; DV = 0.2%; Serving size: 1 small fillet, 170 g

Shrimp Cake Or Patty ☛ Vitamin K = 28.9 mcg; DV = 24.1%; Serving size: 1 cake or patty, 120 g

Shrimp Cocktail ☛ Vitamin K = 4.1 mcg; DV = 3.4%; Serving size: 1 cup, 230 g

Shrimp Creole ☛ Vitamin K = 15.5 mcg; DV = 12.9%; Serving size: 1 cup, 246 g

Shrimp Curry ☛ Vitamin K = 117.5 mcg; DV = 97.9%; Serving size: 1 cup, 236 g

Shrimp Garden Salad With Lettuce And Vegetables ☛ Vitamin K = 61.6 mcg; DV = 51.3%; Serving size: 1 cup, 95 g

Shrimp Gumbo ☛ Vitamin K = 21.7 mcg; DV = 18.1%; Serving size: 1 cup, 244 g

Shrimp In Garlic Sauce Puerto Rican Style ☛ Vitamin K = 94.1 mcg; DV = 78.4%; Serving size: 1 cup, 212 g

Shrimp Mixed Species Raw, Steamed or Boiled ☛ Vitamin K = 0 mcg; DV = 0%; Serving size: 1 medium, 6 g

Shrimp Salad ☛ Vitamin K = 75.3 mcg; DV = 62.8%; Serving size: 1 cup, 182 g

Shrimp Scampi ☛ Vitamin K = 40.7 mcg; DV = 33.9%; Serving size: 1 cup, 136 g

Shrimp Toast Fried ☛ Vitamin K = 14.8 mcg; DV = 12.3%; Serving size: 1/2 slice, 48 g

Shrimp With Crab Stuffing ☛ Vitamin K = 7.8 mcg; DV = 6.5%; Serving size: 1 cup, 140 g

Shrimp With Lobster Sauce ☛ Vitamin K = 8.1 mcg; DV = 6.8%; Serving size: 1 cup, 185 g

Shrimp, Coated Fried (Prepared without Fat) ☛ Vitamin K = 0.4 mcg; DV = 0.3%; Serving size: 1 oz (without shell, cooked), 28 g

Shrimp, Coated Fried (With Oil or Margarine) ☛ Vitamin K = 3.4 mcg; DV = 2.8%; Serving size: 1 oz (without shell, cooked), 28 g

Shrimp, Cooked with Fat (average value) ☛ Vitamin K = 0.1 mcg; DV = 0.1%; Serving size: 1 tiny shrimp, 1 g

Shrimp, Cooked without Fat (average value) ☛ Vitamin K = 0 mcg; DV = 0%; Serving size: 1 tiny shrimp, 1 g

Smelt Rainbow Raw ☛ Vitamin K = 0.1 mcg; DV = 0.1%; Serving size: 3 oz, 85 g

Snapper Mixed Species Raw ☛ Vitamin K = 0.1 mcg; DV = 0.1%; Serving size: 3 oz, 85 g

Squid, Coated Fried (With Oil or Margarine) ☛ Vitamin K = 3.3 mcg; DV = 2.8%; Serving size: 1 oz, cooked, 28 g

Squid, Cooked with Fat (average value) ☛ Vitamin K = 19.6 mcg; DV = 16.3%; Serving size: 1 squid, 272 g

Squid, Cooked with Fat (average value) ☛ Vitamin K = 19.3 mcg; DV = 16.1%; Serving size: 1 squid, 272 g

Squid, Raw, Steamed or Boiled ☛ Vitamin K = 0 mcg; DV = 0%; Serving size: 1 oz, boneless, 28.4 g

Sticks Frozen Prepared ☞ Vitamin K = 2.7 mcg; DV = 2.3%; Serving size: 1 piece, 57 g

Sturgeon, Coated Fried (With Oil or Margarine) ☞ Vitamin K = 3.1 mcg; DV = 2.6%; Serving size: 1 oz, boneless, raw, 27 g

Sturgeon, Cooked without Fat (average value) ☞ Vitamin K = 1 mcg; DV = 0.8%; Serving size: 1 oz, boneless, 23 g

Sturgeon, Cooked without Fat (average value) ☞ Vitamin K = 0 mcg; DV = 0%; Serving size: 1 oz, 28.4 g

Swordfish, Coated Fried (With Oil or Margarine) ☞ Vitamin K = 19.4 mcg; DV = 16.2%; Serving size: 1 small fillet, 170 g

Swordfish, Cooked with Fat (average value) ☞ Vitamin K = 12.1 mcg; DV = 10.1%; Serving size: 1 small fillet, 170 g

Swordfish, Cooked without Fat (average value) ☞ Vitamin K = 7.7 mcg; DV = 6.4%; Serving size: 1 small fillet, 170 g

Tilapia (Raw) ☞ Vitamin K = 1.6 mcg; DV = 1.3%; Serving size: 1 fillet, 116 g

Tilapia, Coated Fried (With Oil or Margarine) ☞ Vitamin K = 14.1 mcg; DV = 11.8%; Serving size: 1 small fillet, 113 g

Tilapia, Coated Fried, Prepared without Fat ☞ Vitamin K = 2.9 mcg; DV = 2.4%; Serving size: 1 small fillet, 113 g

Tilapia, Cooked with Fat (average value) ☞ Vitamin K = 8.1 mcg; DV = 6.8%; Serving size: 1 small fillet, 113 g

Tilapia, Cooked without Fat (average value) ☞ Vitamin K = 2.3 mcg; DV = 1.9%; Serving size: 1 small fillet, 113 g

Trout Smoked ☞ Vitamin K = 0.1 mcg; DV = 0.1%; Serving size: 1 oz, boneless, 28 g

Trout, Cooked with Fat (average value) ☞ Vitamin K = 8 mcg; DV = 6.7%; Serving size: 1 small fillet, 113 g

Trout, Cooked without Fat (average value) ☛ Vitamin K = 0.5 mcg; DV = 0.4%; Serving size: 1 small fillet, 113 g

Tuna And Rice With Mushroom Sauce ☛ Vitamin K = 23.1 mcg; DV = 19.3%; Serving size: 1 cup, 248 g

Tuna Cake Or Patty ☛ Vitamin K = 28.7 mcg; DV = 23.9%; Serving size: 1 cake or patty, 120 g

Tuna Fresh Smoked, Steamed or Poached ☛ Vitamin K = 0 mcg; DV = 0%; Serving size: 1 oz, boneless, 28 g

Tuna Fresh, Cooked with Fat (average value) ☛ Vitamin K = 12.6 mcg; DV = 10.5%; Serving size: 1 small fillet, 170 g

Tuna Fresh, Cooked without Fat (average value) ☛ Vitamin K = 7.7 mcg; DV = 6.4%; Serving size: 1 small fillet, 170 g

Tuna Loaf ☛ Vitamin K = 44 mcg; DV = 36.7%; Serving size: 1 slice, 105 g

Tuna Pot Pie ☛ Vitamin K = 20 mcg; DV = 16.7%; Serving size: 1/8 pie, 96 g

Tuna Salad (average value) ☛ Vitamin K = 96.9 mcg; DV = 80.8%; Serving size: 1 cup, 238 g

Tuna, Canned In Oil ☛ Vitamin K = 64.2 mcg; DV = 53.5%; Serving size: 1 cup, solid or chunks, 146 g

Tuna, Canned In Water ☛ Vitamin K = 0.1 mcg; DV = 0.1%; Serving size: 1 oz, 28.4 g

Turtle Green Raw ☛ Vitamin K = 0.1 mcg; DV = 0.1%; Serving size: 3 oz, 85 g

Whitefish (Raw) ☛ Vitamin K = 0.1 mcg; DV = 0.1%; Serving size: 3 oz, 85 g

Whiting Raw, Steamed Or Poached ☛ Vitamin K = 0.1 mcg; DV = 0.1%; Serving size: 1 fillet, 92 g

Whiting, Coated Fried (With Oil or Margarine) ☛ Vitamin K = 12.9 mcg; DV = 10.8%; Serving size: 1 small fillet, 113 g

Whiting, Cooked with Fat (average value) ☛ Vitamin K = 8 mcg; DV = 6.7%; Serving size: 1 small fillet, 113 g

Whiting, Cooked without Fat (average value) ☛ Vitamin K = 0.5 mcg; DV = 0.4%; Serving size: 1 small fillet, 113 g

FRUITS AND FRUITS PRODUCTS

Acerola Juice, Raw ☞ Vitamin K = 3.4 mcg; DV = 2.8%; Serving size: 1 cup, 242 g

Ambrosia ☞ Vitamin K = 0.6 mcg; DV = 0.5%; Serving size: 1 cup, 193 g

Apple Chips ☞ Vitamin K = 5.2 mcg; DV = 4.3%; Serving size: 1 cup, 28 g

Apple Fried ☞ Vitamin K = 9.3 mcg; DV = 7.8%; Serving size: 1 cup, 179 g

Apple Juice ☞ Vitamin K = 0 mcg; DV = 0%; Serving size: 1 cup, 248 g

Apple Pickled ☞ Vitamin K = 0.4 mcg; DV = 0.3%; Serving size: 1 apple, 29 g

Apple Raw, Baked, Pickled, or Candied ☞ Vitamin K = 3.9 mcg; DV = 3.3%; Serving size: 1 apple with liquid, 161 g

Apple Rings Fried ☞ Vitamin K = 6.9 mcg; DV = 5.8%; Serving size: 5 ring, 85 g

Apples Without Skin ☛ Vitamin K = 0.7 mcg; DV = 0.6%; Serving size: 1 cup slices, 110 g

Applesauce, Canned, Sweetened ☛ Vitamin K = 1.5 mcg; DV = 1.3%; Serving size: 1 cup, 246 g

Apricots Dried ☛ Vitamin K = 2.8 mcg; DV = 2.3%; Serving size: 1 cup, halves, 250 g

Apricots, Raw, Fresh, Frozen or Canned (average value) ☛ Vitamin K = 3.4 mcg; DV = 2.8%; Serving size: 1 cup, halves, 155 g

Asian Pears ☛ Vitamin K = 5.5 mcg; DV = 4.6%; Serving size: 1 fruit, 122 g

Avocados ☛ Vitamin K = 31.5 mcg; DV = 26.3%; Serving size: 1 cup, cubes, 150 g

Banana Batter-Dipped Fried ☛ Vitamin K = 17.7 mcg; DV = 14.8%; Serving size: 1 small, 108 g

Banana Dwarf Fried (Puerto Rican Style) ☛ Vitamin K = 3.7 mcg; DV = 3.1%; Serving size: 1 banana, 36 g

Banana Red, or Rip Fried ☛ Vitamin K = 7.2 mcg; DV = 6%; Serving size: 1 fruit (7-1/4" long), 94 g

Bananas ☛ Vitamin K = 1.1 mcg; DV = 0.9%; Serving size: 1 cup, mashed, 225 g

Bananas Green Pickled Puerto Rican Style ☛ Vitamin K = 27 mcg; DV = 22.5%; Serving size: 1 cup, 150 g

Bartlett Pears ☛ Vitamin K = 5.3 mcg; DV = 4.4%; Serving size: 1 cup, sliced, 140 g

Blackberries Fresh or Frozen ☛ Vitamin K = 28.5 mcg; DV = 23.8%; Serving size: 1 cup, 144 g

Blackberries, Canned ☛ Vitamin K = 34 mcg; DV = 28.3%; Serving size: 1 cup, 256 g

Blackberry Juice, Canned or Fresh ☞ Vitamin K = 38 mcg; DV = 31.7%; Serving size: 1 cup, 250 g

Blueberries Dried ☞ Vitamin K = 23.8 mcg; DV = 19.8%; Serving size: 1/4 cup, 40 g

Blueberries Fresh, Frozen, or Canned (average value) ☞ Vitamin K = 28.6 mcg; DV = 23.8%; Serving size: 1 cup, 148 g

Bosc Pear ☞ Vitamin K = 7.3 mcg; DV = 6.1%; Serving size: 1 cup, sliced, 140 g

Boysenberries Fresh, or Frozen ☞ Vitamin K = 10.3 mcg; DV = 8.6%; Serving size: 1 cup, unthawed, 132 g

Breadfruit ☞ Vitamin K = 1.1 mcg; DV = 0.9%; Serving size: 1 cup, 220 g

California Avocados ☞ Vitamin K = 48.3 mcg; DV = 40.3%; Serving size: 1 cup, pureed, 230 g

Cantaloupe Melons ☞ Vitamin K = 4.4 mcg; DV = 3.7%; Serving size: 1 cup, balls, 177 g

Casaba Melon ☞ Vitamin K = 4.3 mcg; DV = 3.6%; Serving size: 1 cup, cubes, 170 g

Cherries Mixed Species (average value) ☞ Vitamin K = 2.9 mcg; DV = 2.4%; Serving size: 1 cup, with pits, yields, 138 g

Clementines ☞ Vitamin K = 0 mcg; DV = 0%; Serving size: 1 fruit, 74 g

Corn Relish ☞ Vitamin K = 11.8 mcg; DV = 9.8%; Serving size: 1 cup, 245 g

Cranberries ☞ Vitamin K = 5.5 mcg; DV = 4.6%; Serving size: 1 cup, chopped, 110 g

Cranberries Died ☞ Vitamin K = 3 mcg; DV = 2.5%; Serving size: 1/4 cup, 40 g

Cranberry Juice ☛ Vitamin K = 12.9 mcg; DV = 10.8%; Serving size: 1 cup, 253 g

Dates (Deglet Noor) ☛ Vitamin K = 4 mcg; DV = 3.3%; Serving size: 1 cup, chopped, 147 g

Dates Medjool ☛ Vitamin K = 0.6 mcg; DV = 0.5%; Serving size: 1 date, pitted, 24 g

Feijoa ☛ Vitamin K = 8.5 mcg; DV = 7.1%; Serving size: 1 cup, pureed, 243 g

Figs ☛ Vitamin K = 3 mcg; DV = 2.5%; Serving size: 1 large, 64 g

Figs Dried ☛ Vitamin K = 23.2 mcg; DV = 19.3%; Serving size: 1 cup, 149 g

Figs, Canned (average value) ☛ Vitamin K = 13.7 mcg; DV = 11.4%; Serving size: 1 cup, 259 g

Florida Oranges ☛ Vitamin K = 0 mcg; DV = 0%; Serving size: 1 cup sections, without membranes, 185 g

Fruit Cocktail (Peach, Pineapple, Pear, Grape And Cherry) ☛ Vitamin K = 8.9 mcg; DV = 7.4%; Serving size: 1 cup, 248 g

Fruit Juice, Green Machine naked smoothie ☛ Vitamin K = 58.3 mcg; DV = 48.6%; Serving size: 1 cup, 275 g

Fruit Juice, Smoothie Bolthouse Farms Green Goodness ☛ Vitamin K = 18.6 mcg; DV = 15.5%; Serving size: 1 cup, 230 g

Fruit Juice, Smoothie Bolthouse Farms Strawberry Banana ☛ Vitamin K = 2.1 mcg; DV = 1.8%; Serving size: 1 cup, 233 g

Fruit Juice, Smoothie Naked Juice (Strawberry And Banana) ☛ Vitamin K = 4.8 mcg; DV = 4%; Serving size: 1 cup, 228 g

Fruit Juice, Smoothie Odwalla ☛ Vitamin K = 11.4 mcg; DV = 9.5%; Serving size: 1 cup, 227 g

Fruit Salad, Including Citrus Fruits With Salad ☛ Vitamin K = 64.3 mcg; DV = 53.6%; Serving size: 1 cup, 188 g

Fuji Apples ☛ Vitamin K = 1.1 mcg; DV = 0.9%; Serving size: 1 cup, sliced, 109 g

Fuyu Persimmon ☛ Vitamin K = 4.4 mcg; DV = 3.7%; Serving size: 1 fruit, 168 g

Gala Apples ☛ Vitamin K = 1.4 mcg; DV = 1.2%; Serving size: 1 cup, sliced, 109 g

Golden Delicious Apples ☛ Vitamin K = 2 mcg; DV = 1.7%; Serving size: 1 cup, sliced, 109 g

Golden Seedless Raisins ☛ Vitamin K = 5.8 mcg; DV = 4.8%; Serving size: 1 cup, packed, 165 g

Granny Smith Apples ☛ Vitamin K = 3.5 mcg; DV = 2.9%; Serving size: 1 cup, sliced, 109 g

Grape Juice ☛ Vitamin K = 1 mcg; DV = 0.8%; Serving size: 1 cup, 253 g

Grapefruit ☛ Vitamin K = 0 mcg; DV = 0%; Serving size: 1 cup sections, with juice, 230 g

Grapefruit Pink ☛ Vitamin K = 0 mcg; DV = 0%; Serving size: 1 cup sections, with juice, 230 g

Grapefruit White ☛ Vitamin K = 0 mcg; DV = 0%; Serving size: 1 cup sections, with juice, 230 g

Grapes ☛ Vitamin K = 13.4 mcg; DV = 11.2%; Serving size: 1 cup, 92 g

Green Anjou Pear ☛ Vitamin K = 6 mcg; DV = 5%; Serving size: 1 cup, sliced, 140 g

Green Olives ☛ Vitamin K = 0 mcg; DV = 0%; Serving size: 1 olive, 2.7 g

Guanabana Nectar Canned ☛ Vitamin K = 0 mcg; DV = 0%; Serving size: 1 cup, 251 g

Guava Nectar ☛ Vitamin K = 3.4 mcg; DV = 2.8%; Serving size: fl oz, 335 g

Guavas ☛ Vitamin K = 4.3 mcg; DV = 3.6%; Serving size: 1 cup, 165 g

Honeydew Melon ☛ Vitamin K = 4.9 mcg; DV = 4.1%; Serving size: 1 cup, diced (20 pieces per cup), 170 g

Jumbo Olives ☛ Vitamin K = 0.2 mcg; DV = 0.2%; Serving size: 1 super colossal, 15 g

Kiwifruit ☛ Vitamin K = 72.5 mcg; DV = 60.4%; Serving size: 1 cup, sliced, 180 g

Kumquat ☛ Vitamin K = 0 mcg; DV = 0%; Serving size: 1 kumquat, 14 g

Lemon Juice ☛ Vitamin K = 0 mcg; DV = 0%; Serving size: 1 tbsp, 15 g

Lemon Peel Raw ☛ Vitamin K = 0 mcg; DV = 0%; Serving size: 1 tbsp, 6 g

Lemons ☛ Vitamin K = 0 mcg; DV = 0%; Serving size: 1 cup, sections, 212 g

Lime Juice ☛ Vitamin K = 1.5 mcg; DV = 1.3%; Serving size: 1 cup, 242 g

Limes ☛ Vitamin K = 0.4 mcg; DV = 0.3%; Serving size: 1 fruit, 67 g

Litchis ☛ Vitamin K = 0.8 mcg; DV = 0.7%; Serving size: 1 cup, 190 g

Litchis Dried ☛ Vitamin K = 0 mcg; DV = 0%; Serving size: 1 fruit, 2.5 g

Loganberries Fresh or Frozen ☛ Vitamin K = 11.5 mcg; DV = 9.6%; Serving size: 1 cup, unthawed, 147 g

Lychee Fresh, Frozen or Cooked ☞ Vitamin K = 0.1 mcg; DV = 0.1%; Serving size: 1 lychee with liquid, 21 g

Mango Pickled ☞ Vitamin K = 0.8 mcg; DV = 0.7%; Serving size: 1 slice, 28 g

Mangos ☞ Vitamin K = 6.9 mcg; DV = 5.8%; Serving size: 1 cup pieces, 165 g

Mulberries ☞ Vitamin K = 10.9 mcg; DV = 9.1%; Serving size: 1 cup, 140 g

Nance Fresh, Frozen ☞ Vitamin K = 13.3 mcg; DV = 11.1%; Serving size: 1 cup without pits, thawed, 112 g

Naranjilla Pulp, Fresh or Frozen ☞ Vitamin K = 17.5 mcg; DV = 14.6%; Serving size: 1 cup thawed, 120 g

Navel Oranges ☞ Vitamin K = 0 mcg; DV = 0%; Serving size: 1 cup sections, without membranes, 165 g

Nectarines ☞ Vitamin K = 3.1 mcg; DV = 2.6%; Serving size: 1 cup slices, 143 g

Olives All Varieties ☞ Vitamin K = 0 mcg; DV = 0%; Serving size: 1 slice, 1 g

Orange Juice ☞ Vitamin K = 0.2 mcg; DV = 0.2%; Serving size: 1 cup, 248 g

Papaya Dried ☞ Vitamin K = 2 mcg; DV = 1.7%; Serving size: 1 strip, 23 g

Papaya Fresh, Frozen Canned or Cooked ☞ Vitamin K = 3.8 mcg; DV = 3.2%; Serving size: 1 cup, 145 g

Papaya Nectar ☞ Vitamin K = 2 mcg; DV = 1.7%; Serving size: 1 cup, 250 g

Passion Fruit or Granadilla ☞ Vitamin K = 1.7 mcg; DV = 1.4%; Serving size: 1 cup, 236 g

Passion Fruit Purple Juice ☞ Vitamin K = 1 mcg; DV = 0.8%; Serving size: 1 cup, 247 g

Passion Fruit Yellow Juice ☞ Vitamin K = 1 mcg; DV = 0.8%; Serving size: 1 cup, 247 g

Peach Pickled ☞ Vitamin K = 1.6 mcg; DV = 1.3%; Serving size: 1 fruit, 88 g

Peaches Dried ☞ Vitamin K = 25.1 mcg; DV = 20.9%; Serving size: 1 cup, halves, 160 g

Peaches Dried ☞ Vitamin K = 12.9 mcg; DV = 10.8%; Serving size: 1 cup, 258 g

Peaches Fresh, Frozen or Canned (average value) ☞ Vitamin K = 5.5 mcg; DV = 4.6%; Serving size: 1 cup, thawed, 250 g

Peaches Yellow ☞ Vitamin K = 4 mcg; DV = 3.3%; Serving size: 1 cup slices, 154 g

Pear Nectar ☞ Vitamin K = 4.5 mcg; DV = 3.8%; Serving size: 1 cup, 250 g

Pears ☞ Vitamin K = 6.2 mcg; DV = 5.2%; Serving size: 1 cup, slices, 140 g

Pears Dried ☞ Vitamin K = 36.7 mcg; DV = 30.6%; Serving size: 1 cup, halves, 180 g

Pears Dried ☞ Vitamin K = 25.2 mcg; DV = 21%; Serving size: 1 cup, halves, 255 g

Pineapple Dried ☞ Vitamin K = 0.6 mcg; DV = 0.5%; Serving size: 1 piece, 28 g

Pineapple Fresh, Frozen or Canned ☞ Vitamin K = 1.2 mcg; DV = 1%; Serving size: 1 cup, chunks, 165 g

Pineapple Juice ☞ Vitamin K = 2.5 mcg; DV = 2.1%; Serving size: 1 cup, 250 g

Plantains ☛ Vitamin K = 42.6 mcg; DV = 35.5%; Serving size: 1 cup, sliced, 148 g

Plantains Cooked ☛ Vitamin K = 25.8 mcg; DV = 21.5%; Serving size: 1 cup, mashed, 200 g

Plum Pickled ☛ Vitamin K = 1.2 mcg; DV = 1%; Serving size: 1 plum, 28 g

Plums Dried ☛ Vitamin K = 64.7 mcg; DV = 53.9%; Serving size: 1 cup, pitted, 248 g

Plums Fresh, Frozen Or Canned ☛ Vitamin K = 10.6 mcg; DV = 8.8%; Serving size: 1 cup, sliced, 165 g

Pomegranate Juice ☛ Vitamin K = 25.9 mcg; DV = 21.6%; Serving size: 1 cup, 249 g

Pomegranate Raw ☛ Vitamin K = 14.3 mcg; DV = 11.9%; Serving size: 1/2 cup arils (seed/juice sacs), 87 g

Raisins Fresh, or Frozen ☛ Vitamin K = 5.8 mcg; DV = 4.8%; Serving size: 1 cup, packed, 165 g

Raspberries Fresh or Frozen ☛ Vitamin K = 9.6 mcg; DV = 8%; Serving size: 1 cup, 123 g

Red And White Currants ☛ Vitamin K = 12.3 mcg; DV = 10.3%; Serving size: 1 cup, 112 g

Red Anjou Pears ☛ Vitamin K = 6.2 mcg; DV = 5.2%; Serving size: 1 small, 126 g

Red Delicious Apples ☛ Vitamin K = 2.8 mcg; DV = 2.3%; Serving size: 1 cup, sliced, 109 g

Red Or Green Grapes ☛ Vitamin K = 22 mcg; DV = 18.3%; Serving size: 1 cup, 151 g

Rhubarb Cooked Or Canned ☛ Vitamin K = 50.6 mcg; DV = 42.2%; Serving size: 1 cup, 240 g

Rhubarb Fresh or Frozen ☛ Vitamin K = 35.7 mcg; DV = 29.8%; Serving size: 1 cup, diced, 122 g

Seaweed Pickled ☛ Vitamin K = 13.5 mcg; DV = 11.3%; Serving size: 1 cup, 150 g

Starfruit (Carambola) ☛ Vitamin K = 0 mcg; DV = 0%; Serving size: 1 cup, cubes, 132 g

Strawberries Frozen ☛ Vitamin K = 4.9 mcg; DV = 4.1%; Serving size: 1 cup, thawed, 221 g

Strawberries Raw or Frozen ☛ Vitamin K = 3.3 mcg; DV = 2.8%; Serving size: 1 cup, halves, 152 g

Tamarinds ☛ Vitamin K = 3.4 mcg; DV = 2.8%; Serving size: 1 cup, pulp, 120 g

Tangerine Juice ☛ Vitamin K = 0 mcg; DV = 0%; Serving size: 1 cup, 247 g

Tangerines ☛ Vitamin K = 0 mcg; DV = 0%; Serving size: 1 cup, sections, 195 g

Watermelon ☛ Vitamin K = 0.2 mcg; DV = 0.2%; Serving size: 1 cup, balls, 154 g

Yellow Plantains Fried ☛ Vitamin K = 53.7 mcg; DV = 44.8%; Serving size: 1 cup, 169 g

GRAINS AND PASTA

Pasta, Whole Wheat ☞ Vitamin K = 0.7 mcg; DV = 0.6%; Serving size: 1 cup spaghetti, 117 g

Amaranth Grain Uncooked ☞ Vitamin K = 0 mcg; DV = 0%; Serving size: 1 cup, 193 g

Barley, Cooked with Fat ☞ Vitamin K = 3.6 mcg; DV = 3%; Serving size: 1 cup, cooked, 170 g

Barley, Cooked without Fat ☞ Vitamin K = 1.4 mcg; DV = 1.2%; Serving size: 1 cup, cooked, 170 g

Barley Flour, Hulled, Malt flour or Pearled Raw ☞ Vitamin K = 4 mcg; DV = 3.3%; Serving size: 1 cup, 184 g

Buckwheat Flour Whole-Groat ☞ Vitamin K = 8.4 mcg; DV = 7%; Serving size: 1 cup, 120 g

Buckwheat Groats, Cooked with Fat ☞ Vitamin K = 10.9 mcg; DV = 9.1%; Serving size: 1 cup, cooked, 170 g

Buckwheat Groats, Cooked without Fat ☞ Vitamin K = 3.2 mcg; DV = 2.7%; Serving size: 1 cup, cooked, 170 g

Bulgur, Cooked with Fat ☛ Vitamin K = 9.9 mcg; DV = 8.3%; Serving size: 1 cup, cooked, 140 g

Bulgur, Cooked without Fat ☛ Vitamin K = 0.7 mcg; DV = 0.6%; Serving size: 1 cup, cooked, 140 g

Bulgur Dry ☛ Vitamin K = 2.7 mcg; DV = 2.3%; Serving size: 1 cup, 140 g

Congee ☛ Vitamin K = 0 mcg; DV = 0%; Serving size: 1 cup, 249 g

Corn Flour White or Yellow (average value) ☛ Vitamin K = 0 mcg; DV = 0%; Serving size: 1 cup, 114 g

Corn Grain White or Yellow (average value) ☛ Vitamin K = 0.5 mcg; DV = 0.4%; Serving size: 1 cup, 166 g

Cornmeal, Degermed, White or Yellow (average value) ☛ Vitamin K = 0 mcg; DV = 0%; Serving size: 1 cup, 157 g

Cornstarch ☛ Vitamin K = 0 mcg; DV = 0%; Serving size: 1 cup, 128 g

Couscous Plain Cooked ☛ Vitamin K = 0.2 mcg; DV = 0.2%; Serving size: 1 cup, cooked, 157 g

Egg Noodles, Cooked ☛ Vitamin K = 0 mcg; DV = 0%; Serving size: 1 cup, 160 g

Millet, Cooked with Fat ☛ Vitamin K = 9.4 mcg; DV = 7.8%; Serving size: 1 cup, cooked, 170 g

Millet, Cooked without Fat ☛ Vitamin K = 0.5 mcg; DV = 0.4%; Serving size: 1 cup, cooked, 170 g

Millet Flour ☛ Vitamin K = 1 mcg; DV = 0.8%; Serving size: 1 cup, 119 g

Noodles Chinese Chow Mein ☛ Vitamin K = 1.5 mcg; DV = 1.3%; Serving size: 1/2 cup dry, 28 g

Noodles Cooked (average value) ☛ Vitamin K = 0.8 mcg; DV = 0.7%; Serving size: 1 cup, cooked, 160 g

Noodles Vegetable Cooked ☛ Vitamin K = 160.8 mcg; DV = 134%; Serving size: 1 cup, cooked, 160 g

Oat Bran ☛ Vitamin K = 3 mcg; DV = 2.5%; Serving size: 1 cup, 94 g

Oat Flour ☛ Vitamin K = 3.3 mcg; DV = 2.8%; Serving size: 1 cup, 104 g

Oatmeal, Cooked ☛ Vitamin K = 0.7 mcg; DV = 0.6%; Serving size: 1 cup, 234 g

Pasta, Cooked (average value) ☛ Vitamin K = 0.8 mcg; DV = 0.7%; Serving size: 1 cup, cooked, 140 g

Pasta, Gluten-Free (average value) ☛ Vitamin K = 0.5 mcg; DV = 0.4%; Serving size: 1 cup spaghetti not packed, 169 g

Quinoa, Cooked with Fat ☛ Vitamin K = 8.5 mcg; DV = 7.1%; Serving size: 1 cup, cooked, 170 g

Quinoa, Cooked without Fat ☛ Vitamin K = 0 mcg; DV = 0%; Serving size: 1 cup, cooked, 170 g

Rice, Bran ☛ Vitamin K = 2.2 mcg; DV = 1.8%; Serving size: 1 cup, 118 g

Rice, Brown And Wild, Cooked with Fat ☛ Vitamin K = 4.7 mcg; DV = 3.9%; Serving size: 1 cup, cooked, 155 g

Rice, Brown And Wild, Cooked without Fat ☛ Vitamin K = 0.3 mcg; DV = 0.3%; Serving size: 1 cup, cooked, 151 g

Rice, Brown, Cooked with Fat (Butter) ☛ Vitamin K = 0.8 mcg; DV = 0.7%; Serving size: 1 cup, cooked, 196 g

Rice, Brown Cooked with Fat(Margarine) ☛ Vitamin K = 5.1 mcg; DV = 4.3%; Serving size: 1 cup, cooked, 196 g

Rice, Brown Cooked with Fat (Oil) ☛ Vitamin K = 5.7 mcg; DV = 4.8%; Serving size: 1 cup, cooked, 196 g

Rice, Brown Long-Grain Raw ☞ Vitamin K = 1.1 mcg; DV = 0.9%; Serving size: 1 cup, 185 g

Rice, Brown Parboiled Cooked ☞ Vitamin K = 0.6 mcg; DV = 0.5%; Serving size: 1 cup, 155 g

Rice, Flour White ☞ Vitamin K = 0 mcg; DV = 0%; Serving size: 1 cup, 158 g

Rice, Noodles, Cooked ☞ Vitamin K = 0 mcg; DV = 0%; Serving size: 1 cup, 176 g

Rye Grain, Flour Dark, Flour Light or Flour Medium ☞ Vitamin K = 7.6 mcg; DV = 6.3%; Serving size: 1 cup, 128 g

Spaghetti Spinach Dry ☞ Vitamin K = 86.4 mcg; DV = 72%; Serving size: 2 oz, 57 g

Spelt Uncooked ☞ Vitamin K = 6.3 mcg; DV = 5.3%; Serving size: 1 cup, 174 g

Spinach Egg Noodles, Cooked ☞ Vitamin K = 161.8 mcg; DV = 134.8%; Serving size: 1 cup, 160 g

Tapioca Pearl Dry ☞ Vitamin K = 0 mcg; DV = 0%; Serving size: 1 cup, 152 g

Teff Uncooked ☞ Vitamin K = 3.7 mcg; DV = 3.1%; Serving size: 1 cup, 193 g

Wheat Bran Crude ☞ Vitamin K = 1.1 mcg; DV = 0.9%; Serving size: 1 cup, 58 g

Wheat Flour White, Hard White (average value) ☞ Vitamin K = 1.4 mcg; DV = 1.2%; Serving size: 1 cup, 125 g

Wheat Kamut Khorasan ☞ Vitamin K = 3.3 mcg; DV = 2.8%; Serving size: 1 cup, 186 g

Wheat Soft White ☞ Vitamin K = 3.2 mcg; DV = 2.7%; Serving size: 1 cup, 168 g

Rice White ☛ Vitamin K = 0 mcg; DV = 0%; Serving size: 1 cup, 158 g

Whole Grain Sorghum Flour ☛ Vitamin K = 7.7 mcg; DV = 6.4%; Serving size: 1 cup, 121 g

Rice Yellow Cooked with Fat ☛ Vitamin K = 4.1 mcg; DV = 3.4%; Serving size: 1 cup, cooked, 163 g

Rice Yellow Cooked without Fat ☛ Vitamin K = 0.3 mcg; DV = 0.3%; Serving size: 1 cup, cooked, 158 g

MEATS

Armadillo, Cooked ☞ Vitamin K = 0.4 mcg; DV = 0.3%; Serving size: 1 oz, boneless, 28 g

Bacon, And Beef Sticks ☞ Vitamin K = 0.4 mcg; DV = 0.3%; Serving size: 1 oz, 28 g

Bacon, Turkey ☞ Vitamin K = 1.6 mcg; DV = 1.3%; Serving size: 1 serving, 15 g

Bear, Cooked ☞ Vitamin K = 0.5 mcg; DV = 0.4%; Serving size: 1 oz, boneless, 28 g

Beaver, Cooked ☞ Vitamin K = 0.4 mcg; DV = 0.3%; Serving size: 1 oz, boneless, 28 g

Beef, Baloney (Bologna) ☞ Vitamin K = 0.7 mcg; DV = 0.6%; Serving size: 1 slice, 30 g

Beef, Bottom Sirloin, Cooked, (average value) ☞ Vitamin K = 1 mcg; DV = 0.8%; Serving size: 3 oz, 85 g

Beef, Brisket, Lean and Fat, Cooked, (average value) ☞ Vitamin K = 1.5 mcg; DV = 1.3%; Serving size: 3 oz, 85 g

Beef, Burgundy ☞ Vitamin K = 15.6 mcg; DV = 13%; Serving size: 1 cup, 244 g

Beef, Chuck Arm Pot Roast, Cooked, (average value) ☞ Vitamin K = 1.5 mcg; DV = 1.3%; Serving size: 3 oz, 85 g

Beef, Chuck Blade Roast, Cooked, (average value) ☞ Vitamin K = 4.7 mcg; DV = 3.9%; Serving size: 1 piece, 235 g

Beef, Chuck Eye Country-Style Ribs Boneless, Cooked (average value) ☞ Vitamin K = 1.4 mcg; DV = 1.2%; Serving size: 3 oz, 85 g

Beef, Chuck Eye Roast Boneless Americas Beef, Cooked (average value) ☞ Vitamin K = 1.4 mcg; DV = 1.2%; Serving size: 3 oz, 85 g

Beef, Chuck Eye Steak Boneless, Cooked (average value) ☞ Vitamin K = 1.4 mcg; DV = 1.2%; Serving size: 3 oz, 85 g

Beef, Chuck Mock Tender Steak Boneless, Cooked (average value) ☞ Vitamin K = 1.3 mcg; DV = 1.1%; Serving size: 3 oz, 85 g

Beef, Chuck Short Ribs Boneless, Cooked (average value) ☞ Vitamin K = 1.3 mcg; DV = 1.1%; Serving size: 3 oz, 85 g

Beef, Composite Of, Trimmed Retail Cuts, Cooked (average value) ☞ Vitamin K = 1.3 mcg; DV = 1.1%; Serving size: 3 oz, 85 g

Beef, Cow Head, Cooked (average value) ☞ Vitamin K = 0.4 mcg; DV = 0.3%; Serving size: 1 oz, boneless, 28 g

Beef, Flank Steak, Cooked (average value) ☞ Vitamin K = 1.2 mcg; DV = 1%; Serving size: 3 oz, 85 g

Beef, Goulash ☞ Vitamin K = 4 mcg; DV = 3.3%; Serving size: 1 cup, 249 g

Beef, Ground , Cooked (average value) ☞ Vitamin K = 1.5 mcg; DV = 1.3%; Serving size: 3 oz, 85 g

Beef, Liver Braised ☞ Vitamin K = 78.2 mcg; DV = 65.2%; Serving size: 3 oz, 85 g

Beef, Loin Bottom Sirloin Butt Tri-Tip Roast, Cooked (average value) ☞ Vitamin K = 1.1 mcg; DV = 0.9%; Serving size: 1 serving, 85 g

Beef, Loin Tenderloin Roast Boneless, Cooked (average value) ☞ Vitamin K = 1.4 mcg; DV = 1.2%; Serving size: 3 oz, 85 g

Beef, Loin Tenderloin Steak Boneless, Cooked (average value) ☞ Vitamin K = 1.4 mcg; DV = 1.2%; Serving size: 3 oz, 85 g

Beef, Neck Bones, Cooked ☞ Vitamin K = 0.2 mcg; DV = 0.2%; Serving size: 1 oz, with bone, 11 g

Beef, Oxtails, Cooked ☞ Vitamin K = 0.3 mcg; DV = 0.3%; Serving size: 1 oz, with bone, 16 g

Beef, Rib Back Ribs Bone-In, Cooked (average value) ☞ Vitamin K = 1.4 mcg; DV = 1.2%; Serving size: 3 oz, 85 g

Beef, Roast Roasted, Lean Only Eaten ☞ Vitamin K = 0.4 mcg; DV = 0.3%; Serving size: 1 thin slice, 21 g

Beef, Round Bottom Round Roast, Cooked (average value) ☞ Vitamin K = 1.1 mcg; DV = 0.9%; Serving size: 3 oz, 85 g

Beef, Round Tip Round Roast, Cooked (average value) ☞ Vitamin K = 1.1 mcg; DV = 0.9%; Serving size: 3 oz, 85 g

Beef, Sausage ☞ Vitamin K = 0.7 mcg; DV = 0.6%; Serving size: 1 patty, 35 g

Beef, Shortribs, Cooked ☞ Vitamin K = 0.7 mcg; DV = 0.6%; Serving size: 1 small rib, 28 g

Bockwurst Pork Veal, Raw ☞ Vitamin K = 63.9 mcg; DV = 53.3%; Serving size: 1 sausage, 91 g

Chicken Breast, Baked Broiled Or Roasted With Marinade ☞ Vitamin K = 3.9 mcg; DV = 3.3%; Serving size: 1 cup, diced, 135 g

Chicken Breast, Tenders Breaded, Uncooked ☞ Vitamin K = 2.2 mcg; DV = 1.8%; Serving size: 1 piece, 15 g

Chicken Wings, Boneless ☛ Vitamin K = 2.2 mcg; DV = 1.8%; Serving size: 1 boneless wing, 35 g

Chicken, Back ☛ Vitamin K = 5.4 mcg; DV = 4.5%; Serving size: 1 small back, 110 g

Chicken, Canned, Meat Only With Broth ☛ Vitamin K = 2.6 mcg; DV = 2.2%; Serving size: 1 can (5 oz), 142 g

Chicken, Capons, Meat and Skin, Raw ☛ Vitamin K = 2 mcg; DV = 1.7%; Serving size: 3 oz, 85 g

Chicken, Drumstick, Baked Broiled Or Roasted ☛ Vitamin K = 4.3 mcg; DV = 3.6%; Serving size: 1 cup, diced, 135 g

Chicken, Fillet, Grilled ☛ Vitamin K = 4.8 mcg; DV = 4%; Serving size: 1 fillet, 100 g

Chicken, Leg Drumstick And Thigh, Cooked (average value) ☛ Vitamin K = 8.5 mcg; DV = 7.1%; Serving size: 1 cup, diced, 135 g

Chicken, Liver, Fried ☛ Vitamin K = 0.3 mcg; DV = 0.3%; Serving size: 1 oz, raw, 19 g

Chicken, Neck Or Ribs ☛ Vitamin K = 1.4 mcg; DV = 1.2%; Serving size: 1 neck, 35 g

Chicken, Nuggets (average value) ☛ Vitamin K = 1.8 mcg; DV = 1.5%; Serving size: 1 nugget, 16 g

Chicken, Patty Frozen ☛ Vitamin K = 6.7 mcg; DV = 5.6%; Serving size: 1 patty, 60 g

Chicken, Roasting Dark Meat (average value) ☛ Vitamin K = 2.7 mcg; DV = 2.3%; Serving size: 1 unit, 113 g

Chicken, Stewing, Meat And Skin ☛ Vitamin K = 1.7 mcg; DV = 1.4%; Serving size: 3 oz, 85 g

Chicken, Tenders Or Strips Breaded ☛ Vitamin K = 5.5 mcg; DV = 4.6%; Serving size: 1 tender, strip, or finger, 50 g

Chicken, Thigh (average value) ☛ Vitamin K = 7.2 mcg; DV = 6%; Serving size: 1 cup, diced, 135 g

Chicken, Wing, Baked Or Broiled From Fast Food / Restaurant ☛ Vitamin K = 0.9 mcg; DV = 0.8%; Serving size: 1 wing, 35 g

Chicken, Wing, Fried Coated From Pre-Cooked ☛ Vitamin K = 5.3 mcg; DV = 4.4%; Serving size: 1 wing, any size, 55 g

Chicken, Wing, Fried Coated From, Raw ☛ Vitamin K = 4.7 mcg; DV = 3.9%; Serving size: 1 wing, any size, 55 g

Chuck Steak (Mock Tender) ☛ Vitamin K = 2.3 mcg; DV = 1.9%; Serving size: 1 steak, 141 g

Cornish Game Hen, Cooked (average value) ☛ Vitamin K = 7.3 mcg; DV = 6.1%; Serving size: 1 hen (1-1/4 lb, raw), 305 g

Deer Chop, Cooked ☛ Vitamin K = 1 mcg; DV = 0.8%; Serving size: 1 oz, with bone, 23 g

Dove, Cooked ☛ Vitamin K = 5.6 mcg; DV = 4.7%; Serving size: 1 cup, chopped or diced, 140 g

Duck, Cooked (average value) ☛ Vitamin K = 19.4 mcg; DV = 16.2%; Serving size: 1/2 Duck—(yield after cooking, bone removed), 380 g

Frankfurter (average value) ☛ Vitamin K = 1 mcg; DV = 0.8%; Serving size: 1 frankfurter, 57 g

Game Meat Bear, Cooked ☛ Vitamin K = 1.5 mcg; DV = 1.3%; Serving size: 3 oz, 85 g

Game Meat Beaver, Cooked ☛ Vitamin K = 1.4 mcg; DV = 1.2%; Serving size: 3 oz, 85 g

Game Meat Caribou, Cooked ☛ Vitamin K = 1.2 mcg; DV = 1%; Serving size: 3 oz, 85 g

Game Meat Deer Ground, Cooked ☛ Vitamin K = 1 mcg; DV = 0.8%; Serving size: 1 patty (cooked from 4 oz raw), 85 g

Game Meat Opossum, Cooked ☛ Vitamin K = 1.4 mcg; DV = 1.2%; Serving size: 3 oz, 85 g

Game Meat Rabbit, Cooked ☛ Vitamin K = 1.4 mcg; DV = 1.2%; Serving size: 3 oz, 85 g

Game Meat Raccoon, Cooked ☛ Vitamin K = 1.4 mcg; DV = 1.2%; Serving size: 3 oz, 85 g

Game Meat Squirrel, Cooked ☛ Vitamin K = 1.2 mcg; DV = 1%; Serving size: 3 oz, 85 g

Goat Cooked ☛ Vitamin K = 0.3 mcg; DV = 0.3%; Serving size: 1 oz, boneless, 28 g

Goose Domesticated or Wild Cooked ☛ Vitamin K = 7.1 mcg; DV = 5.9%; Serving size: 1 cup, chopped or diced, 140 g

Ham, Breaded Or Floured Fried, Lean And Fat Eaten ☛ Vitamin K = 1.1 mcg; DV = 0.9%; Serving size: 1 thin slice, 21 g

Ham, Croquette ☛ Vitamin K = 14.8 mcg; DV = 12.3%; Serving size: 1 croquette, 62 g

Ham, Fried ☛ Vitamin K = 1.3 mcg; DV = 1.1%; Serving size: 1 thin slice, 21 g

Ham, Or Pork Salad ☛ Vitamin K = 80.6 mcg; DV = 67.2%; Serving size: 1 cup, 182 g

Ham, Stroganoff ☛ Vitamin K = 20 mcg; DV = 16.7%; Serving size: 1 cup, 244 g

Italian Sausage ☛ Vitamin K = 1.2 mcg; DV = 1%; Serving size: 1 patty, 35 g

Lamb, Ground Or Patty, Cooked ☛ Vitamin K = 4.1 mcg; DV = 3.4%; Serving size: 1 patty (4 oz, raw), 77 g

Lamb, Loin Chop, Cooked ☛ Vitamin K = 3.4 mcg; DV = 2.8%; Serving size: 1 small (4 oz, with bone, raw), 71 g

Lamb, Or Mutton Goulash ☛ Vitamin K = 8 mcg; DV = 6.7%; Serving size: 1 cup, 249 g

Lamb, Or Mutton Loaf ☛ Vitamin K = 9.8 mcg; DV = 8.2%; Serving size: 1 small or thin slice, 86 g

Lamb, Ribs, Cooked ☛ Vitamin K = 2.4 mcg; DV = 2%; Serving size: 1 rib, 46 g

Lamb, Roast, Cooked ☛ Vitamin K = 0.6 mcg; DV = 0.5%; Serving size: 1 thin slice, 14 g

Lamb, Shoulder Chop, Cooked ☛ Vitamin K = 4.6 mcg; DV = 3.8%; Serving size: 1 small (5.5 oz, with bone, raw), 100 g

Meatballs, Frozen Italian or Puerto Rican Style ☛ Vitamin K = 7 mcg; DV = 5.8%; Serving size: 3 oz, 85 g

Meatballs, Puerto Rican Style ☛ Vitamin K = 4.4 mcg; DV = 3.7%; Serving size: 1 meatball with sauce, 50 g

Moose, Cooked ☛ Vitamin K = 0.3 mcg; DV = 0.3%; Serving size: 1 oz, boneless, 28 g

Mortadella Beef Pork ☛ Vitamin K = 0.5 mcg; DV = 0.4%; Serving size: 1 oz, 28.4 g

Ostrich, Cooked ☛ Vitamin K = 1 mcg; DV = 0.8%; Serving size: 1 oz, 28 g

Pepperoni ☛ Vitamin K = 4.9 mcg; DV = 4.1%; Serving size: 3 oz, 85 g

Pheasant, Cooked ☛ Vitamin K = 6.4 mcg; DV = 5.3%; Serving size: 1/2 pheasant breast, 130 g

Pork, Bratwurst ☛ Vitamin K = 2.9 mcg; DV = 2.4%; Serving size: 1 link cooked, 85 g

Pork, Chop Cooked ☛ Vitamin K = 1.9 mcg; DV = 1.6%; Serving size: 1 small or thin cut (3 oz, with bone, raw), 52 g

Pork, Ground Or Patty Breaded, Cooked ☛ Vitamin K = 2.4 mcg; DV = 2%; Serving size: 1 oz, raw, 25 g

Pork, Hash ☛ Vitamin K = 27.2 mcg; DV = 22.7%; Serving size: 1 cup, 190 g

Pork, Roll Cured Fried ☛ Vitamin K = 0.4 mcg; DV = 0.3%; Serving size: 1 slice (1 oz), 28 g

Pork, Sausage, Cooked ☛ Vitamin K = 0.9 mcg; DV = 0.8%; Serving size: 1 patty, 30 g

Pork, Steak Or Cutlet Cooked ☛ Vitamin K = 0.4 mcg; DV = 0.3%; Serving size: 1 oz, with bone, raw, 18 g

Pork, Tenderloin Battered Cooked ☛ Vitamin K = 0.6 mcg; DV = 0.5%; Serving size: 1 oz, boneless, raw, 25 g

Quail, Cooked ☛ Vitamin K = 3.2 mcg; DV = 2.7%; Serving size: 1 quail, 75 g

Salami, Cooked Beef ☛ Vitamin K = 0.3 mcg; DV = 0.3%; Serving size: 1 slice, 26 g

Salami, Cooked Beef And Pork ☛ Vitamin K = 0.4 mcg; DV = 0.3%; Serving size: 1 slice round, 12.3 g

Squirrel, Cooked ☛ Vitamin K = 0.3 mcg; DV = 0.3%; Serving size: 1 oz, with bone, 23 g

Turkey, All Classes Back, Cooked (average value) ☛ Vitamin K = 6.7 mcg; DV = 5.6%; Serving size: 1 cup, chopped or diced, 140 g

Turkey, Nuggets ☛ Vitamin K = 2.7 mcg; DV = 2.3%; Serving size: 1 nugget, 20 g

Turkey, Tetrazzini Frozen Meal ☛ Vitamin K = 21.6 mcg; DV = 18%; Serving size: 1 meal (10 oz), 284 g

Veal, Chop, Cooked (average value) ☛ Vitamin K = 4.3 mcg; DV = 3.6%; Serving size: 1 small chop (4.75 oz, with bone, raw), 78 g

Veal, Composite Of Trimmed Retail Cuts, Cooked (average value) ☞ Vitamin K = 5.6 mcg; DV = 4.7%; Serving size: 3 oz, 85 g

Veal, Cordon Bleu ☞ Vitamin K = 64.3 mcg; DV = 53.6%; Serving size: 1 roll, 229 g

Veal, Cutlet Or Steak Broiled, Cooked (average value) ☞ Vitamin K = 1.5 mcg; DV = 1.3%; Serving size: 1 oz, boneless, 28 g

Veal, Foreshank Osso Buco, Cooked (average value) ☞ Vitamin K = 1.3 mcg; DV = 1.1%; Serving size: 3 oz, 85 g

Veal, Fricassee, Puerto Rican Style ☞ Vitamin K = 11.3 mcg; DV = 9.4%; Serving size: 1 cup, 230 g

Veal, Ground Or Patty, Cooked ☞ Vitamin K = 0.6 mcg; DV = 0.5%; Serving size: 1 small patty (3.2 oz, raw, 5 patties per lb), 54 g

Veal, Leg (Top Round), Cooked (average value) ☞ Vitamin K = 6 mcg; DV = 5%; Serving size: 3 oz, 85 g

Veal, Loin, Cooked (average value) ☞ Vitamin K = 4.7 mcg; DV = 3.9%; Serving size: 3 oz, 85 g

Veal, Marsala ☞ Vitamin K = 18.7 mcg; DV = 15.6%; Serving size: 1 slice with sauce, 96 g

Veal, Parmigiana ☞ Vitamin K = 10.4 mcg; DV = 8.7%; Serving size: 1 patty with sauce and cheese, 182 g

Veal, Patty Breaded, Cooked ☞ Vitamin K = 3.4 mcg; DV = 2.8%; Serving size: 1 small patty (3.2 oz, raw, 5 patties per lb), 64 g

Veal, Rib, Cooked (average value) ☞ Vitamin K = 6 mcg; DV = 5%; Serving size: 3 oz, 85 g

Veal, Scallopini ☞ Vitamin K = 15 mcg; DV = 12.5%; Serving size: 1 slice with sauce, 96 g

Veal, Shoulder Arm, Cooked (average value) ☞ Vitamin K = 1.3 mcg; DV = 1.1%; Serving size: 1 oz, 28.4 g

Veal, Shoulder Blade, Cooked (average value) ☞ Vitamin K = 5.8 mcg; DV = 4.8%; Serving size: 3 oz, 85 g

Veal, Shoulder Whole (Arm And Blade), Cooked (average value) ☞ Vitamin K = 5 mcg; DV = 4.2%; Serving size: 3 oz, 85 g

Veal, Sirloin, Separable Lean And Fat, Cooked (average value) ☞ Vitamin K = 5.6 mcg; DV = 4.7%; Serving size: 3 oz, 85 g

Venison/deer, Cooked (average value) ☞ Vitamin K = 0.4 mcg; DV = 0.3%; Serving size: 1 oz, boneless, 28 g

NUTS AND SEEDS

Almond Dry, Roasted, Blanched, Butter And Paste ☛ Vitamin K = 0 mcg; DV = 0%; Serving size: 1 tbsp, 16 g

Almonds Honey—Roasted ☛ Vitamin K = 13.5 mcg; DV = 11.3%; Serving size: 1 cup, chopped, 115 g

Almonds Oil ☛ Vitamin K = 0 mcg; DV = 0%; Serving size: 1 cup whole kernels, 157 g

Brazilnuts ☛ Vitamin K = 0 mcg; DV = 0%; Serving size: 1 cup, whole, 133 g

Cashew Butter Plain ☛ Vitamin K = 4.8 mcg; DV = 4%; Serving size: 1 tbsp, 16 g

Cashew Dry, Roasted or Unroasted ☛ Vitamin K = 51 mcg; DV = 42.5%; Serving size: 1 cup, halves and whole, 137 g

Cashew Oil ☛ Vitamin K = 44.8 mcg; DV = 37.3%; Serving size: 1 cup, whole, 129 g

Coconut Dried ☛ Vitamin K = 0.1 mcg; DV = 0.1%; Serving size: 1 oz, 28.4 g

Coconut Milk, Raw ☛ Vitamin K = 0.2 mcg; DV = 0.2%; Serving size: 1 cup, 240 g

Coconut Water ☛ Vitamin K = 0 mcg; DV = 0%; Serving size: 1 cup, 240 g

Flax Seeds ☛ Vitamin K = 0.4 mcg; DV = 0.3%; Serving size: 1 tbsp, whole, 10.3 g

Hazelnuts ☛ Vitamin K = 16.3 mcg; DV = 13.6%; Serving size: 1 cup, chopped, 115 g

Macadamia Nuts, Dry Or Roasted ☛ Vitamin K = 0 mcg; DV = 0%; Serving size: 1 cup, whole or halves, 132 g

Mixed Dry Roasted (average value) ☛ Vitamin K = 19.3 mcg; DV = 16.1%; Serving size: 1 cup, 142 g

Mixed Oil, Roasted (average value) ☛ Vitamin K = 25.8 mcg; DV = 21.5%; Serving size: 1 cup, 144 g

Mixed Seeds ☛ Vitamin K = 4.6 mcg; DV = 3.8%; Serving size: 1 cup, 145 g

Mixed Unroasted (average value) ☛ Vitamin K = 19 mcg; DV = 15.8%; Serving size: 1 cup, 142 g

Oil—Roasted Cashews ☛ Vitamin K = 44.8 mcg; DV = 37.3%; Serving size: 1 cup, whole, 129 g

Peanut Butter ☛ Vitamin K = 0 mcg; DV = 0%; Serving size: 1 tablespoon, 16 g

Peanuts Dry—Roasted ☛ Vitamin K = 0 mcg; DV = 0%; Serving size: 1 cup, 146 g

Pecans Honey—Roasted ☛ Vitamin K = 15.3 mcg; DV = 12.8%; Serving size: 1 cup, chopped, 109 g

Pecans, Salted or Unsalted ☛ Vitamin K = 7.5 mcg; DV = 6.3%; Serving size: 1 cup, chopped, 109 g

Pine Dried ☞ Vitamin K = 72.8 mcg; DV = 60.7%; Serving size: 1 cup, 135 g

Pistachio Dry, Roasted With or Without Salt (average value) ☞ Vitamin K = 20 mcg; DV = 16.7%; Serving size: 1 cup, 123 g

Pumpkin And Squash Seeds Dried ☞ Vitamin K = 9.4 mcg; DV = 7.8%; Serving size: 1 cup, 129 g

Pumpkin—Salted ☞ Vitamin K = 6.3 mcg; DV = 5.3%; Serving size: 1 cup, without shell, 144 g

Chestnuts Roasted ☞ Vitamin K = 11.2 mcg; DV = 9.3%; Serving size: 1 cup, 143 g

Squash And Pumpkin, Roasted ☞ Vitamin K = 5.3 mcg; DV = 4.4%; Serving size: 1 cup, 118 g

Sesame Butter Tahini ☞ Vitamin K = 0 mcg; DV = 0%; Serving size: 1 tbsp, 15 g

Sesame Seed Kernels Dried Or Toasted ☞ Vitamin K = 0 mcg; DV = 0%; Serving size: 1 cup, 150 g

Sesame Whole Dried ☞ Vitamin K = 0 mcg; DV = 0%; Serving size: 1 cup, 144 g

Sunflower Dry—Roasted ☞ Vitamin K = 3.5 mcg; DV = 2.9%; Serving size: 1 cup, 128 g

Sunflower Seed Kernels Dry—Roasted ☞ Vitamin K = 3.5 mcg; DV = 2.9%; Serving size: 1 cup, 128 g

Sunflower Seed Kernels Oil ☞ Vitamin K = 4.2 mcg; DV = 3.5%; Serving size: 1 cup, 135 g

Sunflower Seeds Dried ☞ Vitamin K = 0 mcg; DV = 0%; Serving size: 1 cup, with hulls, edible yield, 46 g

Trail Mix—With And Fruit ☞ Vitamin K = 10.8 mcg; DV = 9%; Serving size: 1 cup, 140 g

Trail Mix—With Chocolate ☛ Vitamin K = 10.4 mcg; DV = 8.7%; Serving size: 1 cup, 140 g

Trail Mix—With Nuts ☛ Vitamin K = 13.9 mcg; DV = 11.6%; Serving size: 1 cup, 140 g

Trail Mix—With Pretzels or Cereal ☛ Vitamin K = 9.9 mcg; DV = 8.3%; Serving size: 1 cup, 140 g

Walnuts ☛ Vitamin K = 3.2 mcg; DV = 2.7%; Serving size: 1 cup, chopped, 117 g

PREPARED MEALS

Rice And Vermicelli Mix, Beef Flavor, Unprepared ☛ Vitamin K = 1.5 mcg; DV = 1.3%; Serving size: 1/ 3 cup, 61 g

Almond Chicken ☛ Vitamin K = 30.7 mcg; DV = 25.6%; Serving size: 1 cup, 242 g

Beans String Green Cooked Szechuan-Style ☛ Vitamin K = 105.3 mcg; DV = 87.8%; Serving size: 1 cup, 185 g

Beef And Broccoli ☛ Vitamin K = 135.8 mcg; DV = 113.2%; Serving size: 1 cup, 217 g

Beef And Noodles, With Soy Base Sauce ☛ Vitamin K = 41.3 mcg; DV = 34.4%; Serving size: 1 cup, 249 g

Beef And Rice, With Soy Base Sauce ☛ Vitamin K = 41.5 mcg; DV = 34.6%; Serving size: 1 cup, 244 g

Beef And Vegetables (With Dark-Green Leafy Carrots Broccoli) ☛ Vitamin K = 83.8 mcg; DV = 69.8%; Serving size: 1 cup, 217 g

Beef And Vegetables (Without Dark-Green Leafy Carrots Broccoli) ☛ Vitamin K = 44.7 mcg; DV = 37.3%; Serving size: 1 cup, 217 g

Beef Chow Mein ☞ Vitamin K = 29.3 mcg; DV = 24.4%; Serving size: 1 cup, 220 g

Corned Beef Hash With Potato ☞ Vitamin K = 4.2 mcg; DV = 3.5%; Serving size: 1 cup, 236 g

Beef Enchilada Dinner (Frozen Meal) ☞ Vitamin K = 10.6 mcg; DV = 8.8%; Serving size: 1 meal (15 oz), 425 g

Beef Macaroni ☞ Vitamin K = 7 mcg; DV = 5.8%; Serving size: 1 serving, 269 g

Beef Noodles And Vegetables (With Dark-Green Leafy Carrots Broccoli) ☞ Vitamin K = 71.8 mcg; DV = 59.8%; Serving size: 1 cup, 217 g

Beef Noodles And Vegetables (Without Dark-Green Leafy Carrots Broccoli) ☞ Vitamin K = 38.2 mcg; DV = 31.8%; Serving size: 1 cup, 217 g

Beef Rice And Vegetables (With Dark-Green Leafy Carrots Broccoli) ☞ Vitamin K = 72.9 mcg; DV = 60.8%; Serving size: 1 cup, 217 g

Beef Rice And Vegetables (Without Dark-Green Leafy Carrots Broccoli) ☞ Vitamin K = 38.6 mcg; DV = 32.2%; Serving size: 1 cup, 217 g

Beef Tofu And Vegetables (With Dark-Green Leafy Carrots Broccoli) ☞ Vitamin K = 81.4 mcg; DV = 67.8%; Serving size: 1 cup, 217 g

Beef Tofu And Vegetables (Without Dark-Green Leafy Carrots Broccoli) ☞ Vitamin K = 43.6 mcg; DV = 36.3%; Serving size: 1 cup, 217 g

Beef With Soy Base Sauce ☞ Vitamin K = 50.3 mcg; DV = 41.9%; Serving size: 1 cup, 244 g

Beef With Sweet And Sour Sauce ☞ Vitamin K = 21.2 mcg; DV = 17.7%; Serving size: 1 cup, 252 g

Bibimbap Korean ☞ Vitamin K = 133.8 mcg; DV = 111.5%; Serving size: 1 cup, 162 g

Biryani With Chicken or Meat ☛ Vitamin K = 12.2 mcg; DV = 10.2%; Serving size: 1 cup, 196 g

Biryani, With Vegetables ☛ Vitamin K = 4.8 mcg; DV = 4%; Serving size: 1 cup, 172 g

Burrito Various Combinations (average value) ☛ Vitamin K = 9.8 mcg; DV = 8.2%; Serving size: 1 burrito, 129 g

Cannelloni Cheese- And Spinach-Filled No Sauce ☛ Vitamin K = 75.3 mcg; DV = 62.8%; Serving size: 1 cannelloni, 74 g

Cannelloni Cheese-Filled (No Spinach) ☛ Vitamin K = 2.3 mcg; DV = 1.9%; Serving size: 1 meal (9.125 oz), 259 g

Cheese Enchilada (Frozen Meal) ☛ Vitamin K = 11.9 mcg; DV = 9.9%; Serving size: 1 meal (10 oz), 284 g

Cheese Quiche Meatless ☛ Vitamin K = 6.3 mcg; DV = 5.3%; Serving size: 1 piece, 192 g

Cheese Turnover, Puerto Rican Style ☛ Vitamin K = 1.1 mcg; DV = 0.9%; Serving size: 1 turnover, 21 g

Chicken Chow Mein (Frozen Meal) ☛ Vitamin K = 18.8 mcg; DV = 15.7%; Serving size: 1 lean cuisine meal (11.25 oz), 319 g

Chicken Egg Foo Yung ☛ Vitamin K = 15.9 mcg; DV = 13.3%; Serving size: 1 patty, 86 g

Chicken Enchilada (Frozen Meal) ☛ Vitamin K = 7.2 mcg; DV = 6%; Serving size: 1 meal (8.5 oz), 241 g

Chicken Fajitas (Frozen Meal) ☛ Vitamin K = 5.9 mcg; DV = 4.9%; Serving size: 1 meal (6.75 oz), 191 g

Chicken Or Turkey With Noodles, Or Rice And Soy Base Sauce ☛ Vitamin K = 36.7 mcg; DV = 30.6%; Serving size: 1 cup, 224 g

Chicken Or Turkey (With Dark-Green Leafy Carrots Broccoli) ☛ Vitamin K = 43.6 mcg; DV = 36.3%; Serving size: 1 cup, 217 g

Chicken Tenders Breaded (Frozen) ☞ Vitamin K = 3.7 mcg; DV = 3.1%; Serving size: 1 piece, 21 g

Chilaquiles Tortilla Casserole ☞ Vitamin K = 21.1 mcg; DV = 17.6%; Serving size: 1 cup, 232 g

Chiles Rellenos Cheese-Filled ☞ Vitamin K = 16.4 mcg; DV = 13.7%; Serving size: 1 chili, 143 g

Chili Con Carne ☞ Vitamin K = 11.1 mcg; DV = 9.3%; Serving size: 1 cup, 242 g

Chimichanga Meatless ☞ Vitamin K = 13.1 mcg; DV = 10.9%; Serving size: 1 small chimichanga, 128 g

Chimichanga, With Meat Or Chicken ☞ Vitamin K = 12.1 mcg; DV = 10.1%; Serving size: 1 small chimichanga, 105 g

Dumpling Fried, Puerto Rican Style ☞ Vitamin K = 12 mcg; DV = 10%; Serving size: 1 dumpling, 97 g

Dumpling Meat-Filled ☞ Vitamin K = 9.1 mcg; DV = 7.6%; Serving size: 1 dumpling, any size, 97 g

Dumpling Potato Or Cheese-Filled ☞ Vitamin K = 9 mcg; DV = 7.5%; Serving size: 3 pieces pierogies, 114 g

Dumpling Vegetable ☞ Vitamin K = 30.6 mcg; DV = 25.5%; Serving size: 1 dumpling, any size, 97 g

Egg Rolls Meatless ☞ Vitamin K = 41 mcg; DV = 34.2%; Serving size: 1 egg roll, 89 g

Egg Roll (With Meat, Chicken Or Turkey) ☞ Vitamin K = 27.9 mcg; DV = 23.3%; Serving size: 1 egg roll, 89 g

Egg Roll, With Shrimp ☞ Vitamin K = 41 mcg; DV = 34.2%; Serving size: 1 egg roll, 89 g

Egg Rolls Vegetable (Frozen Prepared) ☞ Vitamin K = 35.1 mcg; DV = 29.3%; Serving size: 1 egg roll, 89 g

Mexican Empanada (Cheese And Vegetables) ☛ Vitamin K = 6.4 mcg; DV = 5.3%; Serving size: 1 small/appetizer, 81 g

Mexican Empanada (Chicken And Vegetables) ☛ Vitamin K = 6 mcg; DV = 5%; Serving size: 1 small/appetizer, 81 g

Enchilada With Cheese Only Meatless ☛ Vitamin K = 11 mcg; DV = 9.2%; Serving size: 1 enchilada, any size, 111 g

Enchilada, With Green Beans ☛ Vitamin K = 13.9 mcg; DV = 11.6%; Serving size: 1 enchilada, any size, 132 g

Enchilada, With Beans Meatless ☛ Vitamin K = 8.3 mcg; DV = 6.9%; Serving size: 1 enchilada, any size, 141 g

Enchilada, With Chicken And Green Beans ☛ Vitamin K = 13.1 mcg; DV = 10.9%; Serving size: 1 enchilada, any size, 132 g

Enchilada, With Chicken And Red-Chile Or Enchilada Sauce ☛ Vitamin K = 4.9 mcg; DV = 4.1%; Serving size: 1 enchilada, any size, 123 g

Fajita, With Vegetables ☛ Vitamin K = 8.6 mcg; DV = 7.2%; Serving size: 1 fajita, 141 g

Fish And Vegetables (With Dark-Green Leafy Carrots Broccoli) ☛ Vitamin K = 82.5 mcg; DV = 68.8%; Serving size: 1 cup, 217 g

Fish And Vegetables (Without Dark-Green Leafy Carrots Broccoli) ☛ Vitamin K = 43.4 mcg; DV = 36.2%; Serving size: 1 cup, 217 g

Fried Stuffed Potatoes, Puerto Rican Style ☛ Vitamin K = 11.3 mcg; DV = 9.4%; Serving size: 1 fritter, 95 g

Gnocchi Cheese ☛ Vitamin K = 4.9 mcg; DV = 4.1%; Serving size: 1 cup, 70 g

Gnocchi Potato ☛ Vitamin K = 2.6 mcg; DV = 2.2%; Serving size: 1 cup, 188 g

Gordita Sope Or Chalupa (average value) ☛ Vitamin K = 16.7 mcg;

DV = 13.9%; Serving size: 1 small, 150 g

Grape Leaves Stuffed, With Rice ☛ Vitamin K = 34.9 mcg; DV = 29.1%; Serving size: 1 roll, 56 g

Knish Cheese ☛ Vitamin K = 11.1 mcg; DV = 9.3%; Serving size: 1 knish, 60 g

Knish Meat ☛ Vitamin K = 8.7 mcg; DV = 7.3%; Serving size: 1 knish, 50 g

Knish Potato ☛ Vitamin K = 12.4 mcg; DV = 10.3%; Serving size: 1 knish, 61 g

Kung Pao Beef, Pork or Shrimp ☛ Vitamin K = 21.7 mcg; DV = 18.1%; Serving size: 1 cup, 162 g

Lasagna, Cheese ☛ Vitamin K = 20.5 mcg; DV = 17.1%; Serving size: 1 cup 1 serving, 225 g

Lasagna, Meatless Spinach Noodles ☛ Vitamin K = 109 mcg; DV = 90.8%; Serving size: 1 piece, 227 g

Lasagna, Meatless Whole Wheat Noodles ☛ Vitamin K = 41.8 mcg; DV = 34.8%; Serving size: 1 piece, 227 g

Lasagna, Meatless, With Vegetables ☛ Vitamin K = 41.8 mcg; DV = 34.8%; Serving size: 1 piece, 227 g

Lasagna, Vegetable ☛ Vitamin K = 40.4 mcg; DV = 33.7%; Serving size: 1 serving, 227 g

Lasagna, With Meat Spinach Noodles ☛ Vitamin K = 70.7 mcg; DV = 58.9%; Serving size: 1 piece, 206 g

Lasagna, With Meat Whole Wheat Noodles ☛ Vitamin K = 10.1 mcg; DV = 8.4%; Serving size: 1 piece, 206 g

Linguini, With Vegetables And Seafood ☛ Vitamin K = 47.6 mcg; DV = 39.7%; Serving size: 1 meal (9.5 oz), 269 g

Lo Mein, With Beef, Chicken or Beef ☛ Vitamin K = 21.2 mcg; DV =

17.7%; Serving size: 1 cup, 200 g

Macaroni And Cheese Box (average value) ☛ Vitamin K = 15.6 mcg; DV = 13%; Serving size: 1 serving, 244 g

Macaroni Or Noodles, With Cheese (average value) ☛ Vitamin K = 11 mcg; DV = 9.2%; Serving size: 1 cup, 230 g

Macaroni Or Pasta Salad Made, With Dressing (Mayonnaise, Italian Dressing, Creaming Dressing) ☛ Vitamin K = 56.5 mcg; DV = 47.1%; Serving size: 1 cup, 204 g

Macaroni Or Pasta Salad With Meat, Crab, Shrimp, Tuna, Chicken (average value) ☛ Vitamin K = 47.7 mcg; DV = 39.8%; Serving size: 1 cup, 204 g

Manicotti Cheese-Filled ☛ Vitamin K = 2.5 mcg; DV = 2.1%; Serving size: 1 manicotti, 127 g

Manicotti Vegetable And Cheese-Filled, Meatless ☛ Vitamin K = 46.6 mcg; DV = 38.8%; Serving size: 1 manicotti, 143 g

Meat Turnover, Puerto Rican Style ☛ Vitamin K = 13.3 mcg; DV = 11.1%; Serving size: 5 turnover, 140 g

Mexican Casserole ☛ Vitamin K = 8.2 mcg; DV = 6.8%; Serving size: 1 cup, 144 g

Moo Goo Gai Pan ☛ Vitamin K = 33.5 mcg; DV = 27.9%; Serving size: 1 cup, 216 g

Moo Shu Pork, Without Chinese ☛ Vitamin K = 52.7 mcg; DV = 43.9%; Serving size: 1 cup, 151 g

Nachos, With Cheese, Chicken, Chili Or Meat And Sour Cream ☛ Vitamin K = 0.4 mcg; DV = 0.3%; Serving size: 1 nacho, 7 g

Pad Thai Meatless ☛ Vitamin K = 41 mcg; DV = 34.2%; Serving size: 1 cup, 200 g

Pad Thai With Chicken, Meat Or Seafood (average value) ☛ Vitamin

K = 38.2 mcg; DV = 31.8%; Serving size: 1 cup, 200 g

Paella (average value) ☛ Vitamin K = 12.2 mcg; DV = 10.2%; Serving size: 1 cup, 240 g

Pasta Meat-Filled ☛ Vitamin K = 6.3 mcg; DV = 5.3%; Serving size: 1 cup, 250 g

Pasta Mix, Classic Beef ☛ Vitamin K = 0.4 mcg; DV = 0.3%; Serving size: 1 package, 122 g

Pasta Mix, Italian Lasagna ☛ Vitamin K = 18.2 mcg; DV = 15.2%; Serving size: 1 package, 141 g

Pasta, With Tomato Based Sauce And Seafood ☛ Vitamin K = 32.8 mcg; DV = 27.3%; Serving size: 1 cup, 250 g

Pasta, With Tomato-Based Sauce Restaurant ☛ Vitamin K = 35.8 mcg; DV = 29.8%; Serving size: 1 cup, 250 g

Pasta, With Vegetables Without Sauce Or Dressing ☛ Vitamin K = 30.9 mcg; DV = 25.8%; Serving size: 1 cup, 150 g

Pizza Rolls, Frozen ☛ Vitamin K = 3.7 mcg; DV = 3.1%; Serving size: 1 serving 6 rolls, 80 g

Pork And Onions With Soy Base Sauce ☛ Vitamin K = 36.9 mcg; DV = 30.8%; Serving size: 1 cup, 256 g

Pork And Vegetables Hawaiian Style ☛ Vitamin K = 40.8 mcg; DV = 34%; Serving size: 1 cup, 252 g

Pork And Vegetables (With Dark-Green Leafy, Carrots Broccoli) ☛ Vitamin K = 82.7 mcg; DV = 68.9%; Serving size: 1 cup, 217 g

Pork And Vegetables (Without Dark-Green Leafy, Carrots Broccoli) ☛ Vitamin K = 43.6 mcg; DV = 36.3%; Serving size: 1 cup, 217 g

Pork And Watercress With Soy Base Sauce ☛ Vitamin K = 198 mcg; DV = 165%; Serving size: 1 cup, 162 g

Pork Chow Mein Or Chop Suey With or Without Noodles ☛ Vitamin

K = 27.9 mcg; DV = 23.3%; Serving size: 1 cup, 220 g

Pork Egg Foo Yung ☛ Vitamin K = 15.6 mcg; DV = 13%; Serving size: 1 patty, 86 g

Pork Or Ham, With Soy Base Sauce ☛ Vitamin K = 48.6 mcg; DV = 40.5%; Serving size: 1 cup, 244 g

Pork Rice And Vegetables (With Dark-Green Leafy, Carrots Broccoli) ☛ Vitamin K = 71.8 mcg; DV = 59.8%; Serving size: 1 cup, 217 g

Pork Rice And Vegetables (Without Dark-Green Leafy, Carrots Broccoli) ☛ Vitamin K = 37.8 mcg; DV = 31.5%; Serving size: 1 cup, 217 g

Pork Tofu And Vegetables (With Dark-Green Leafy, Carrots Broccoli) ☛ Vitamin K = 80.7 mcg; DV = 67.3%; Serving size: 1 cup, 217 g

Pork Tofu And Vegetables (Without Dark-Green Leafy, Carrots Broccoli) ☛ Vitamin K = 43 mcg; DV = 35.8%; Serving size: 1 cup, 217 g

Potato And Ham Fritters (Puerto Rican Style) ☛ Vitamin K = 10.4 mcg; DV = 8.7%; Serving size: 1 fritter, 70 g

Potato Mashed From Dry Mix (average value) ☛ Vitamin K = 9.3 mcg; DV = 7.8%; Serving size: 1 cup, 250 g

Potato Mashed, From Fast Food ☛ Vitamin K = 12 mcg; DV = 10%; Serving size: 1 cup, 250 g

Potato Mashed From Fresh (average value) ☛ Vitamin K = 3.8 mcg; DV = 3.2%; Serving size: 1 cup, 250 g

Potato Mashed From Restaurant ☛ Vitamin K = 8.5 mcg; DV = 7.1%; Serving size: 1 cup, 250 g

Potato Pancake ☛ Vitamin K = 1.2 mcg; DV = 1%; Serving size: 1 miniature/bite size pancake, 10 g

Potato Pudding ☛ Vitamin K = 10.5 mcg; DV = 8.8%; Serving size: 1 cup, 228 g

Potato Salad Made, With Creamy Dressing ☛ Vitamin K = 69.6 mcg;

DV = 58%; Serving size: 1 cup, 275 g

Potato Salad Made, With Italian Dressing ☛ Vitamin K = 33 mcg; DV = 27.5%; Serving size: 1 cup, 275 g

Potato Salad Made With Mayonnaise ☛ Vitamin K = 76.5 mcg; DV = 63.8%; Serving size: 1 cup, 275 g

Potato Salad, From Restaurant ☛ Vitamin K = 76.5 mcg; DV = 63.8%; Serving size: 1 cup, 275 g

Potato Salad, With Egg ☛ Vitamin K = 17.9 mcg; DV = 14.9%; Serving size: 1/2 cup, 125 g

Potato Salad, With Egg Made And Creamy Dressing ☛ Vitamin K = 61.1 mcg; DV = 50.9%; Serving size: 1 cup, 275 g

Potato Salad, With Egg Made And Italian Dressing ☛ Vitamin K = 29.2 mcg; DV = 24.3%; Serving size: 1 cup, 275 g

Potato Salad, With Egg Made, With Light Mayonnaise ☛ Vitamin K = 30 mcg; DV = 25%; Serving size: 1 cup, 275 g

Pork Potsticker Or Wonton With Vegetable ☛ Vitamin K = 79.8 mcg; DV = 66.5%; Serving size: 5 pieces 1 serving, 145 g

Quesadilla, With Chicken Or Meat And Vegetables (average value) ☛ Vitamin K = 2.1 mcg; DV = 1.8%; Serving size: 1 slice or wedge, 20 g

Ravioli, Cheese And Spinach Filled, With Tomato Sauce ☛ Vitamin K = 97.3 mcg; DV = 81.1%; Serving size: 4 piece, 152 g

Ravioli, Cheese And Spinach-Filled ☛ Vitamin K = 104.4 mcg; DV = 87%; Serving size: 8 piece, 120 g

Ravioli, Cheese And Spinach-Filled, With Cream Sauce ☛ Vitamin K = 94.8 mcg; DV = 79%; Serving size: 4 piece, 152 g

Ravioli, Cheese-Filled ☛ Vitamin K = 5.6 mcg; DV = 4.7%; Serving size: 1 cup, 242 g

Ravioli, Cheese-Filled No Sauce ☛ Vitamin K = 0.6 mcg; DV = 0.5%;

Serving size: 8 piece, 120 g

Ravioli, Cheese-Filled, With Cream Sauce ☛ Vitamin K = 5.9 mcg; DV = 4.9%; Serving size: 4 piece, 152 g

Ravioli, Cheese-Filled, With Meat Sauce ☛ Vitamin K = 4.6 mcg; DV = 3.8%; Serving size: 4 piece, 140 g

Ravioli, Cheese-Filled, With Tomato Sauce ☛ Vitamin K = 21.6 mcg; DV = 18%; Serving size: 4 piece, 152 g

Red Beans And Rice ☛ Vitamin K = 17.5 mcg; DV = 14.6%; Serving size: 1 cup, 224 g

Rice Croquette ☛ Vitamin K = 38.1 mcg; DV = 31.8%; Serving size: 1 croquette , 124 g

Rice Fried, With Beef, Pork, Shrimp Or Chicken (average value) ☛ Vitamin K = 5.1 mcg; DV = 4.3%; Serving size: 1 cup, 198 g

Rice Meal Fritter, Puerto Rican Style ☛ Vitamin K = 6.6 mcg; DV = 5.5%; Serving size: 5 cruller, 150 g

Rice, With Beans And Beef, Chicken, Or Pork (average value) ☛ Vitamin K = 19.6 mcg; DV = 16.3%; Serving size: 1 cup, 239 g

Rice, With Broccoli Cheese Sauce ☛ Vitamin K = 68.1 mcg; DV = 56.8%; Serving size: 4.5 oz, 128 g

Rice, With Chicken, Puerto Rican Style ☛ Vitamin K = 10.4 mcg; DV = 8.7%; Serving size: 1 cup, 157 g

Rice, With Squid, Puerto Rican Style ☛ Vitamin K = 15.5 mcg; DV = 12.9%; Serving size: 1 cup, 160 g

Rice, With Vienna Sausage, Puerto Rican Style ☛ Vitamin K = 9.2 mcg; DV = 7.7%; Serving size: 1 cup, 180 g

Shrimp And Noodles, With Soy Base Sauce ☛ Vitamin K = 36.3 mcg; DV = 30.3%; Serving size: 1 cup, 224 g

Shrimp And Vegetables (With Dark-Green Leafy, Carrots Broccoli) ☛

Vitamin K = 82.9 mcg; DV = 69.1%; Serving size: 1 cup, 217 g

Shrimp And Vegetables (Without Dark-Green Leafy, Carrots Broccoli) ☛ Vitamin K = 43.8 mcg; DV = 36.5%; Serving size: 1 cup, 217 g

Shrimp Chow Mein With or Without Noodles ☛ Vitamin K = 27.5 mcg; DV = 22.9%; Serving size: 1 cup, 220 g

Shrimp Egg Foo Yung ☛ Vitamin K = 32 mcg; DV = 26.7%; Serving size: 1 cup, 175 g

Soft Taco, With Meat, Fish Or Chicken ☛ Vitamin K = 8.1 mcg; DV = 6.8%; Serving size: 1 small taco or tostada, 103 g

Somen Salad (With Lettuce Egg Fish And Pork) ☛ Vitamin K = 30.9 mcg; DV = 25.8%; Serving size: 1 cup, 160 g

Spaghetti With Tomato Sauce (average value) ☛ Vitamin K = 19.5 mcg; DV = 16.3%; Serving size: 12.5 oz, 354 g

Spanakopitta ☛ Vitamin K = 189.2 mcg; DV = 157.7%; Serving size: 3 pieces, 89 g

Spinach Quiche Meatless ☛ Vitamin K = 163.3 mcg; DV = 136.1%; Serving size: 1 piece, 143 g

Stuffed Shells (Cheese And Spinach) ☛ Vitamin K = 54 mcg; DV = 45%; Serving size: 1 shell, 60 g

Sushi (average value) ☛ Vitamin K = 2.6 mcg; DV = 2.2%; Serving size: 4 piece, 120 g

Tabbouleh ☛ Vitamin K = 161.4 mcg; DV = 134.5%; Serving size: 1 cup, 160 g

Taco Or Tostada Salad (average value) ☛ Vitamin K = 30.4 mcg; DV = 25.3%; Serving size: 1 small taco salad, 234 g

Taco Or Tostada (average value) ☛ Vitamin K = 11 mcg; DV = 9.2%; Serving size: 1 small taco or tostada, 125 g

Taco, With Crab Meat, Puerto Rican Style ☛ Vitamin K = 8 mcg; DV

= 6.7%; Serving size: 1 taco (4-1/2" dia), 121 g

Tamale Casserole, Puerto Rican Style ☛ Vitamin K = 9.7 mcg; DV = 8.1%; Serving size: 1 cup, 237 g

Tamale (average value) ☛ Vitamin K = 4.6 mcg; DV = 3.8%; Serving size: 1 cup, 244 g

Taquitos Beef And Cheese ☛ Vitamin K = 9.2 mcg; DV = 7.7%; Serving size: 1 piece, 42 g

Taquitos, Chicken And Cheese ☛ Vitamin K = 7.1 mcg; DV = 5.9%; Serving size: 1 piece, 42 g

Tofu And Vegetables (With Dark-Green Leafy, Carrots Broccoli) ☛ Vitamin K = 76.4 mcg; DV = 63.7%; Serving size: 1 cup, 217 g

Tofu And Vegetables (Without Dark-Green Leafy, Carrots Broccoli) ☛ Vitamin K = 41 mcg; DV = 34.2%; Serving size: 1 cup, 217 g

Tortellini, Cheese-Filled Meatless, With Vegetables ☛ Vitamin K = 54.6 mcg; DV = 45.5%; Serving size: 1 cup, 169 g

Tortellini, Spinach-Filled No Sauce ☛ Vitamin K = 53.3 mcg; DV = 44.4%; Serving size: 1 cup, 122 g

Tortellini, Spinach-Filled, With Tomato Sauce ☛ Vitamin K = 94.4 mcg; DV = 78.7%; Serving size: 1 cup, 200 g

Vegetable Combination (With Dark-Green Leafy, Carrots Broccoli) ☛ Vitamin K = 104.2 mcg; DV = 86.8%; Serving size: 1 cup, 185 g

Vegetable Combination (Without Dark-Green Leafy, Carrots Broccoli) ☛ Vitamin K = 55.9 mcg; DV = 46.6%; Serving size: 1 cup, 185 g

Wonton Fried Filled (With Meat Poultry Or Seafood And Vegetable) ☛ Vitamin K = 12.2 mcg; DV = 10.2%; Serving size: 1 wonton, any size, 19 g

Wonton Fried Meatless ☛ Vitamin K = 12.2 mcg; DV = 10.2%; Serving size: 1 wonton, any size, 19 g

RESTAURANT FOODS

Applebees—Chicken Tenders (Kids Menu) ☛ Vitamin K = 8.8 mcg; DV =7.3%; Serving size: 1 piece, 35 g

Applebees—Coleslaw ☛ Vitamin K = 49.5 mcg; Serving size: 1 serving, 76 g

Applebees—Double Crunch Shrimp ☛ Vitamin K = 59.9 mcg; Serving size: 1 serving, 206 g

Applebees—French Fries ☛ Vitamin K = 54.8 mcg; Serving size: 1 serving, 164 g

Applebees—Mozzarella Sticks ☛ Vitamin K = 7.1 mcg; Serving size: 1 piece, 32 g

Carrabba's Italian Grill—Spaghetti With Meat Sauce ☛ Vitamin K = 17.7 mcg; Serving size: 1 serving, 537 g

Carrabba's Italian Grill—Spaghetti With Pomodoro Sauce ☛ Vitamin K = 21.5 mcg; Serving size: 1 serving, 489 g

Chinese Restaurant—Beef And Vegetables ☛ Vitamin K = 294.5 mcg; Serving size: 1 order, 574 g

Chinese Restaurant—Chicken And Vegetables ☛ Vitamin K = 379.1 mcg; Serving size: 1 order, 693 g

Chinese Restaurant—Chicken Chow Mein ☛ Vitamin K = 132.9 mcg; Serving size: 1 order, 604 g

Chinese Restaurant—Egg Rolls Assorted ☛ Vitamin K = 52.4 mcg; Serving size: 1 piece, 89 g

Chinese Restaurant—Fried Rice Without Meat ☛ Vitamin K = 3.8 mcg; Serving size: 1 cup, 137 g

Chinese Restaurant—General Tsos Chicken ☛ Vitamin K = 204.4 mcg; Serving size: 1 order, 535 g

Chinese Restaurant—Kung Pao Chicken ☛ Vitamin K = 82.1 mcg; Serving size: 1 order, 604 g

Chinese Restaurant—Lemon Chicken ☛ Vitamin K = 152 mcg; Serving size: 1 order, 623 g

Chinese Restaurant—Orange Chicken ☛ Vitamin K = 158.1 mcg; Serving size: 1 order, 648 g

Chinese Restaurant—Sesame Chicken ☛ Vitamin K = 148.2 mcg; Serving size: 1 order, 547 g

Chinese Restaurant—Shrimp And Vegetables ☛ Vitamin K = 312.5 mcg; Serving size: 1 order, 601 g

Chinese Restaurant—Sweet And Sour Chicken ☛ Vitamin K = 158.9 mcg; Serving size: 1 order, 706 g

Chinese Restaurant—Sweet And Sour Pork ☛ Vitamin K = 169.9 mcg; Serving size: 1 order, 609 g

Chinese Restaurant—Vegetable Chow Mein Without Meat Or Noodles ☛ Vitamin K = 146.9 mcg; Serving size: 1 order, 777 g

Chinese Restaurant—Vegetable Lo Mein Without Meat ☛ Vitamin K = 94.1 mcg; Serving size: 1 order, 741 g

Cracker Barrel—Chicken Tenderloin Platter Fried (Kids Menu) ☞ Vitamin K = 34.3 mcg; Serving size: 1 serving, 103 g

Cracker Barrel—Coleslaw ☞ Vitamin K = 147.1 mcg; Serving size: 1 serving, 167 g

Cracker Barrel—Farm Raised Catfish Platter ☞ Vitamin K = 44 mcg; Serving size: 1 serving, 178 g

Cracker Barrel—Grilled Sirloin Steak ☞ Vitamin K = 1.5 mcg; Serving size: 1 steak, 151 g

Cracker Barrel—Macaroni N Cheese Plate (Kids Menu) ☞ Vitamin K = 25.4 mcg; Serving size: 1 serving, 257 g

Cracker Barrel—Onion Rings Thick-Cut ☞ Vitamin K = 94.2 mcg; Serving size: 1 serving, 261 g

Cracker Barrel—Steak Fries ☞ Vitamin K = 63.6 mcg; Serving size: 1 serving, 198 g

Denny's—Chicken Nuggets Star Shaped (Kids Menu) ☞ Vitamin K = 24.5 mcg; Serving size: 1 serving 4 pieces, 67 g

Denny's—Coleslaw ☞ Vitamin K = 78.4 mcg; Serving size: 1 serving, 91 g

Denny's—French Fries ☞ Vitamin K = 47.5 mcg; Serving size: 1 serving, 165 g

Denny's—Golden Fried Shrimp ☞ Vitamin K = 5.6 mcg; Serving size: 1 piece, 16 g

Denny's—Hash Browns ☞ Vitamin K = 40.4 mcg; Serving size: 1 serving, 124 g

Denny's—Macaroni & Cheese (Kids Menu) ☞ Vitamin K = 5.4 mcg; Serving size: 1 serving, 180 g

Denny's—Mozzarella Cheese Sticks ☞ Vitamin K = 57.9 mcg; Serving size: 1 serving, 228 g

Denny's—Onion Rings ☛ Vitamin K = 84 mcg; Serving size: 1 serving, 166 g

Denny's—Top Sirloin Steak ☛ Vitamin K = 1.1 mcg; Serving size: 1 steak, 107 g

Family Style Restaurant—Chicken Fingers From Kids Menu ☛ Vitamin K = 31.9 mcg; Serving size: 1 serving, 114 g

Family Style Restaurant—Chili With Meat And Beans ☛ Vitamin K = 4.2 mcg; Serving size: 1 cup, 136 g

Family Style Restaurant—Coleslaw ☛ Vitamin K = 85.3 mcg; Serving size: 1 serving, 108 g

Family Style Restaurant—Fish Fillet Battered Or Breaded Fried ☛ Vitamin K = 0.2 mcg; Serving size: 1 serving, 226 g

Family Style Restaurant—French Fries ☛ Vitamin K = 61 mcg; Serving size: 1 serving, 170 g

Family Style Restaurant—Fried Mozzarella Sticks ☛ Vitamin K = 56.1 mcg; Serving size: 1 serving, 245 g

Family Style Restaurant—Hash Browns ☛ Vitamin K = 30.6 mcg; Serving size: 1 cup, 94 g

Family Style Restaurant—Macaroni & Cheese From Kids Menu ☛ Vitamin K = 0.7 mcg; Serving size: 1 cup, 136 g

Family Style Restaurant—Onion Rings ☛ Vitamin K = 110.3 mcg; Serving size: 1 serving, 259 g

Family Style Restaurant—Shrimp Breaded And Fried ☛ Vitamin K = 54.4 mcg; Serving size: 1 serving, 169 g

French Fries ☛ Vitamin K = 1.6 mcg; Serving size: 10 strip, 69 g

Fried Onion Rings ☛ Vitamin K = 143.9 mcg; Serving size: 1 serving, 350 g

Hash Browns ☛ Vitamin K = 5.8 mcg; Serving size: 1 cup, 156 g

Italian Restaurant—Lasagna With Meat ☞ Vitamin K = 31.1 mcg; Serving size: 1 serving, 457 g

Italian Restaurant—Spaghetti With Meat Sauce ☞ Vitamin K = 23.3 mcg; Serving size: 1 serving, 554 g

Italian Restaurant—Spaghetti With Pomodoro Sauce (No Meat) ☞ Vitamin K = 20.4 mcg; Serving size: 1 serving, 510 g

Latino Restaurant—Arepa (Unleavened Cornmeal Bread) ☞ Vitamin K = 3.4 mcg; Serving size: 1 piece, 98 g

Latino Restaurant—Arroz Con Frijoles Negros (Rice And Black Beans) ☞ Vitamin K = 47.5 mcg; Serving size: 1 serving, 461 g

Latino Restaurant—Arroz Con Grandules (Rice And Pigeonpeas) ☞ Vitamin K = 82.3 mcg; Serving size: 1 serving, 653 g

Latino Restaurant—Arroz Con Habichuelas Colorados (Rice And Red Beans) ☞ Vitamin K = 46 mcg; Serving size: 1 serving, 590 g

Latino Restaurant—Black Bean Soup ☞ Vitamin K = 14.8 mcg; Serving size: 1 cup, 246 g

Latino Restaurant—Bunuelos (Fried Yeast Bread) ☞ Vitamin K = 18.1 mcg; Serving size: 1 piece, 70 g

Latino Restaurant—Chicken And Rice Entree Prepared ☞ Vitamin K = 5.6 mcg; Serving size: 1 cup, 141 g

Latino Restaurant—Empanadas Beef Prepared ☞ Vitamin K = 5.4 mcg; Serving size: 1 piece, 89 g

Latino Restaurant—Pupusas Con Frijoles (Pupusas Bean) ☞ Vitamin K = 9.3 mcg; Serving size: 1 piece, 126 g

Latino Restaurant—Pupusas Con Queso (Pupusas Cheese) ☞ Vitamin K = 2 mcg; Serving size: 1 piece, 117 g

Latino Restaurant—Pupusas Del Cerdo (Pupusas Pork) ☞ Vitamin K = 1.3 mcg; Serving size: 1 piece, 122 g

Latino Restaurant—Tamale Corn ☛ Vitamin K = 9 mcg; Serving size: 1 piece, 166 g

Latino Restaurant—Tamale Pork ☛ Vitamin K = 7.2 mcg; Serving size: 1 piece, 142 g

Latino Restaurant—Tripe Soup ☛ Vitamin K = 4.6 mcg; Serving size: 1 cup, 200 g

Mexican Restaurant—Refried Beans ☛ Vitamin K = 19.7 mcg; Serving size: 1 cup, 148 g

Mexican Restaurant—Spanish Rice ☛ Vitamin K = 15.1 mcg; Serving size: 1 cup, 116 g

Olive Garden—Lasagna Classico ☛ Vitamin K = 28.7 mcg; Serving size: 1 serving, 422 g

Olive Garden—Spaghetti With Meat Sauce ☛ Vitamin K = 22.6 mcg; Serving size: 1 serving, 525 g

Olive Garden—Spaghetti With Pomodoro Sauce ☛ Vitamin K = 20.1 mcg; Serving size: 1 serving, 478 g

On The Border—Mexican Rice ☛ Vitamin K = 14 mcg; Serving size: 1 cup, 114 g

On The Border—Refried Beans ☛ Vitamin K = 2.8 mcg; Serving size: 1 cup, 135 g

Onion Rings ☛ Vitamin K = 16.4 mcg; Serving size: 1 cup, 48 g

T.G.I. Friday's—Chicken Fingers (Kids Menu) ☛ Vitamin K = 10.4 mcg; Serving size: 1 piece, 41 g

T.G.I. Friday's—French Fries ☛ Vitamin K = 79.3 mcg; Serving size: 1 serving, 184 g

SPICES AND HERBS

Apple Cider Vinegar ☛ Vitamin K = 0 mcg; DV = 0%; Serving size: 1 tbsp, 14.9 g

Basil ☛ Vitamin K = 10.4 mcg; DV = 8.7%; Serving size: 5 leaves, 2.5 g

Black Pepper ☛ Vitamin K = 3.8 mcg; DV = 3.2%; Serving size: 1 tsp, ground, 2.3 g

Capers ☛ Vitamin K = 2.1 mcg; DV = 1.8%; Serving size: 1 tbsp, drained, 8.6 g

Caraway Seed ☛ Vitamin K = 0 mcg; DV = 0%; Serving size: 1 tsp, 2.1 g

Cayenne Pepper ☛ Vitamin K = 1.4 mcg; DV = 1.2%; Serving size: 1 tsp, 1.8 g

Celery Seed ☛ Vitamin K = 0 mcg; DV = 0%; Serving size: 1 tsp, 2 g

Chili Powder ☛ Vitamin K = 2.9 mcg; DV = 2.4%; Serving size: 1 tsp, 2.7 g

Cinnamon ☛ Vitamin K = 0.8 mcg; DV = 0.7%; Serving size: 1 tsp, 2.6 g

Cumin Seed ☞ Vitamin K = 0.1 mcg; DV = 0.1%; Serving size: 1 tsp, whole, 2.1 g

Curry Powder ☞ Vitamin K = 2 mcg; DV = 1.7%; Serving size: 1 tsp, 2 g

Distilled Vinegar ☞ Vitamin K = 0 mcg; DV = 0%; Serving size: 1 tbsp, 14.9 g

Dried Basil ☞ Vitamin K = 12 mcg; DV = 10%; Serving size: 1 tsp, leaves, 0.7 g

Dried Coriander ☞ Vitamin K = 8.2 mcg; DV = 6.8%; Serving size: 1 tsp, 0.6 g

Dried Marjoram ☞ Vitamin K = 3.7 mcg; DV = 3.1%; Serving size: 1 tsp, 0.6 g

Dried Oregano ☞ Vitamin K = 6.2 mcg; DV = 5.2%; Serving size: 1 tsp, leaves, 1 g

Dried Parsley ☞ Vitamin K = 6.8 mcg; DV = 5.7%; Serving size: 1 tsp, 0.5 g

Garlic Powder ☞ Vitamin K = 0 mcg; DV = 0%; Serving size: 1 tsp, 3.1 g

Ground Cloves ☞ Vitamin K = 3 mcg; DV = 2.5%; Serving size: 1 tsp, 2.1 g

Ground Ginger ☞ Vitamin K = 0 mcg; DV = 0%; Serving size: 1 tsp, 1.8 g

Ground Mustard Seed ☞ Vitamin K = 0.1 mcg; DV = 0.1%; Serving size: 1 tsp, 2 g

Ground Nutmeg ☞ Vitamin K = 0 mcg; DV = 0%; Serving size: 1 tsp, 2.2 g

Ground Sage ☞ Vitamin K = 12 mcg; DV = 10%; Serving size: 1 tsp, 0.7 g

Ground Turmeric ☛ Vitamin K = 0.4 mcg; DV = 0.3%; Serving size: 1 tsp, 3 g

Horseradish ☛ Vitamin K = 0.1 mcg; DV = 0.1%; Serving size: 1 tsp, 5 g

Onion Powder ☛ Vitamin K = 0.1 mcg; DV = 0.1%; Serving size: 1 tsp, 2.4 g

Paprika ☛ Vitamin K = 1.8 mcg; DV = 1.5%; Serving size: 1 tsp, 2.3 g

Poppy Seeds ☛ Vitamin K = 0 mcg; DV = 0%; Serving size: 1 tsp, 2.8 g

Poultry Seasoning ☛ Vitamin K = 12.1 mcg; DV = 10.1%; Serving size: 1 tsp, 1.5 g

Pumpkin Pie Spice ☛ Vitamin K = 0.5 mcg; DV = 0.4%; Serving size: 1 tsp, 1.7 g

Spices Thyme Dried ☛ Vitamin K = 17.1 mcg; DV = 14.3%; Serving size: 1 tsp, leaves, 1 g

Table Salt ☛ Vitamin K = 0 mcg; DV = 0%; Serving size: 1 tsp, 6 g

Vanilla Extract ☛ Vitamin K = 0 mcg; DV = 0%; Serving size: 1 tsp, 4.2 g

Yellow Mustard ☛ Vitamin K = 0.1 mcg; DV = 0.1%; Serving size: 1 tsp or 1 packet, 5 g

SWEETS

Honey ☛ Vitamin K = 0 mcg; DV = 0%; Serving size: 1 cup, 339 g

Molasses ☛ Vitamin K = 0 mcg; DV = 0%; Serving size: 1 cup, 337 g

Sugar ☛ Vitamin K = 0 mcg; DV = 0%; Serving size: 1 serving packet, 2.8 g

Sugar Brown And Water Syrup ☛ Vitamin K = 0 mcg; DV = 0%; Serving size: 1 cup, 242 g

Sugar Brown Liquid ☛ Vitamin K = 0 mcg; DV = 0%; Serving size: 1 cup, 335 g

Sugar Cinnamon ☛ Vitamin K = 4.4 mcg; DV = 3.7%; Serving size: 1 cup, 200 g

Sugar Substitute And Sugar Blend ☛ Vitamin K = 0 mcg; DV = 0%; Serving size: 1 teaspoon, 2 g

Sugar Substitute Liquid Nfs ☛ Vitamin K = 0 mcg; DV = 0%; Serving size: 1 teaspoon, 5 g

Sugar Substitute Powder Nfs ☛ Vitamin K = 0 mcg; DV = 0%; Serving size: 1 individual packet, 1 g

Sugar Substitute Saccharin Liquid ☛ Vitamin K = 0 mcg; DV = 0%; Serving size: 1 teaspoon, 5 g

Sugar Substitute Stevia Liquid ☛ Vitamin K = 0 mcg; DV = 0%; Serving size: 1 teaspoon, 5 g

Sugar White And Water Syrup ☛ Vitamin K = 0 mcg; DV = 0%; Serving size: 1 cup, 242 g

Sugar-Coated Almonds ☛ Vitamin K = 0 mcg; DV = 0%; Serving size: 1 piece, 3.5 g

Sugared Pecans Sugar And Egg White Coating ☛ Vitamin K = 1.9 mcg; DV = 1.6%; Serving size: 1 cup, 79 g

Sugars Brown ☛ Vitamin K = 0 mcg; DV = 0%; Serving size: 1 tsp unpacked, 3 g

Sugars Maple ☛ Vitamin K = 0 mcg; DV = 0%; Serving size: 1 tsp, 3 g

Syrup Cane ☛ Vitamin K = 0 mcg; DV = 0%; Serving size: 1 serving, 21 g

Syrups Maple ☛ Vitamin K = 0 mcg; DV = 0%; Serving size: 1 tbsp, 20 g

VEGETABLES AND VEGETABLES PRODUCTS

Alfalfa Sprouts ☛ Vitamin K = 10.1 mcg; DV = 8.4%; Serving size: 1 cup, 33 g

Amaranth Leaves, Raw ☛ Vitamin K = 319.2 mcg; DV = 266%; Serving size: 1 cup, 28 g

Artichoke Salad In Oil ☛ Vitamin K = 24.1 mcg; DV = 20.1%; Serving size: 1 cup, 130 g

Artichokes Green, Fresh, Frozen Or Canned, Cooked With Fat ☛ Vitamin K = 17.8 mcg; DV = 14.8%; Serving size: 1 artichoke, medium, 120 g

Artichokes Green, Fresh, Frozen Or Canned, Cooked Without Fat ☛ Vitamin K = 15 mcg; DV = 12.5%; Serving size: 1 artichoke, medium, 120 g

Artichokes Green ☛ Vitamin K = 16.4 mcg; DV = 13.7%; Serving size: 1 artichoke, medium, 128 g

Artichokes Stuffed ☛ Vitamin K = 74 mcg; DV = 61.7%; Serving size: 1 stuffed globe, 251 g

Arugula ☛ Vitamin K = 2.2 mcg; DV = 1.8%; Serving size: 1 leaf, 2 g

Asparagus ☛ Vitamin K = 55.7 mcg; DV = 46.4%; Serving size: 1 cup, 134 g

Asparagus Canned, Cooked Without Fat ☛ Vitamin K = 99.5 mcg; DV = 82.9%; Serving size: 1 cup, 242 g

Asparagus Fresh or Frozen, Cooked Without Fat ☛ Vitamin K = 1.5 mcg; DV = 1.3%; Serving size: 1 piece, 3 g

Asparagus, Cooked Boiled, Drained ☛ Vitamin K = 45.5 mcg; DV = 37.9%; Serving size: 1/2 cup, 90 g

Baby Carrots ☛ Vitamin K = 1.4 mcg; DV = 1.2%; Serving size: 1 large, 15 g

Bamboo Shoots ☛ Vitamin K = 0 mcg; DV = 0%; Serving size: 1 cup, 151 g

Bamboo Shoots, Cooked With Fat ☛ Vitamin K = 7.5 mcg; DV = 6.3%; Serving size: 1 cup, 156 g

Bamboo Shoots, Cooked Without Fat ☛ Vitamin K = 0 mcg; DV = 0%; Serving size: 1 cup, slices, 120 g

Banana Peppers ☛ Vitamin K = 11.8 mcg; DV = 9.8%; Serving size: 1 cup, 124 g

Bean Sprouts, Fresh or Frozen, Cooked With Fat ☛ Vitamin K = 59.2 mcg; DV = 49.3%; Serving size: 1 cup, 129 g

Beet Greens, Cooked Boiled, Drained ☛ Vitamin K = 697 mcg; DV = 580.8%; Serving size: 1 cup, 144 g

Beet Greens, Cooked Without Fat ☛ Vitamin K = 692.2 mcg; DV = 576.8%; Serving size: 1 cup, 144 g

Beet Greens, Raw ☛ Vitamin K = 152 mcg; DV = 126.7%; Serving size: 1 cup, 38 g

Beets Cooked, Canned, Without Fat ☛ Vitamin K = 0.3 mcg; DV = 0.3%; Serving size: 1 cup, whole, 163 g

Beets Cooked, Fresh or Frozen, Without Fat ☛ Vitamin K = 0.3 mcg; DV = 0.3%; Serving size: 1 cup, whole, 163 g

Beets, Raw ☛ Vitamin K = 0.3 mcg; DV = 0.3%; Serving size: 1 cup, 136 g

Bitter Melon, Cooked With Fat ☛ Vitamin K = 11.2 mcg; DV = 9.3%; Serving size: 1 cup, 129 g

Bitter Melon, Cooked Without Fat ☛ Vitamin K = 6 mcg; DV = 5%; Serving size: 1 cup, 124 g

Bok Choy ☛ Vitamin K = 31.9 mcg; DV = 26.6%; Serving size: 1 cup, shredded, 70 g

Breadfruit Fried ☛ Vitamin K = 8.7 mcg; DV = 7.3%; Serving size: 1 cup, 170 g

Breadfruit, Cooked With Fat ☛ Vitamin K = 5.1 mcg; DV = 4.3%; Serving size: 1 cup, 257 g

Breadfruit, Cooked Without Fat ☛ Vitamin K = 1.5 mcg; DV = 1.3%; Serving size: 1 cup, 252 g

Broccoflower, Cooked Without Fat ☛ Vitamin K = 17 mcg; DV = 14.2%; Serving size: 1 cup, fresh, 82 g

Broccoli ☛ Vitamin K = 92.5 mcg; DV = 77.1%; Serving size: 1 cup chopped, 91 g

Broccoli Fresh or Frozen, Cooked Without Fat ☛ Vitamin K = 218.7 mcg; DV = 182.3%; Serving size: 1 cup, fresh, cut stalks, 156 g

Broccoli, Cooked Boiled, Drained ☛ Vitamin K = 220.1 mcg; DV = 183.4%; Serving size: 1 cup, fresh, cut stalks, 156 g

Broccoli, Raab ☛ Vitamin K = 89.6 mcg; DV = 74.7%; Serving size: 1 cup chopped, 40 g

Broccoli, Raab, Cooked Without Fat ☛ Vitamin K = 432.7 mcg; DV = 360.6%; Serving size: 1 cup, 170 g

Broccoli, Slaw Salad ☛ Vitamin K = 150.3 mcg; DV = 125.3%; Serving size: 1 cup, 186 g

Brussels Sprouts Fresh or Frozen, Cooked Without Fat ☛ Vitamin K = 216.1 mcg; DV = 180.1%; Serving size: 1 cup, 155 g

Brussels Sprouts, Cooked Boiled, Drained ☛ Vitamin K = 154.8 mcg; DV = 129%; Serving size: 1/2 cup, 80 g

Brussels Sprouts, Fresh or Frozen, Creamed ☛ Vitamin K = 178.3 mcg; DV = 148.6%; Serving size: 1 cup, 228 g

Brussels Sprouts, Raw ☛ Vitamin K = 155.8 mcg; DV = 129.8%; Serving size: 1 cup, 88 g

Burdock Root, Raw ☛ Vitamin K = 1.9 mcg; DV = 1.6%; Serving size: 1 cup, 118 g

Burdock, Cooked With Fat ☛ Vitamin K = 7.8 mcg; DV = 6.5%; Serving size: 1 cup, 130 g

Burdock, Cooked Without Fat ☛ Vitamin K = 2.5 mcg; DV = 2.1%; Serving size: 1 cup, 125 g

Cabbage ☛ Vitamin K = 67.6 mcg; DV = 56.3%; Serving size: 1 cup, chopped, 89 g

Cabbage Chinese, Cooked Boiled, Drained ☛ Vitamin K = 57.8 mcg; DV = 48.2%; Serving size: 1 cup, shredded, 170 g

Cabbage Common, Cooked Boiled, Drained ☛ Vitamin K = 81.5 mcg; DV = 67.9%; Serving size: 1/2 cup, shredded, 75 g

Cabbage Mustard ☛ Vitamin K = 148 mcg; DV = 123.3%; Serving size: 1 cup, 128 g

Cabbage Salad Or Coleslaw, Made With Various Dressing (average value) ☛ Vitamin K = 141 mcg; DV = 117.5%; Serving size: 1 cup, 219 g

Cabbage Salad Or Coleslaw, Made, With Creamy Dressing ☛ Vitamin K = 175 mcg; DV = 145.8%; Serving size: 1 cup, 219 g

Cabbage, Creamed ☛ Vitamin K = 119.2 mcg; DV = 99.3%; Serving size: 1 cup, 200 g

Cactus, Cooked Without Fat ☛ Vitamin K = 7.6 mcg; DV = 6.3%; Serving size: 1 cup, 149 g

Caesar Salad With Romaine, No Dressing ☛ Vitamin K = 70.4 mcg; DV = 58.7%; Serving size: 1 cup, 79 g

Calabaza, Cooked ☛ Vitamin K = 27.4 mcg; DV = 22.8%; Serving size: 1 cup, cubes, 166 g

Candied Ripe Plantain, Puerto Rican Style ☛ Vitamin K = 12.3 mcg; DV = 10.3%; Serving size: 1 serving (1/2 plantain with syrup), 140 g

Carrot Dehydrated ☛ Vitamin K = 79.9 mcg; DV = 66.6%; Serving size: 1 cup, 74 g

Carrots ☛ Vitamin K = 16.9 mcg; DV = 14.1%; Serving size: 1 cup chopped, 128 g

Carrots Cooked, From Canned, Without Fat ☛ Vitamin K = 0.2 mcg; DV = 0.2%; Serving size: 1 baby carrot, 2 g

Carrots Fresh or Frozen, Cooked Without Fat ☛ Vitamin K = 1.2 mcg; DV = 1%; Serving size: 1 baby carrot, 9 g

Carrots, Cooked Boiled, Drained ☛ Vitamin K = 21.4 mcg; DV = 17.8%; Serving size: 1 cup, sliced, 156 g

Carrots, Fresh or Frozen, Creamed ☛ Vitamin K = 18.2 mcg; DV = 15.2%; Serving size: 1 cup, 228 g

Carrots, In Tomato Sauce ☛ Vitamin K = 17.2 mcg; DV = 14.3%; Serving size: 1 cup, 176 g

Cassava ☛ Vitamin K = 3.9 mcg; DV = 3.3%; Serving size: 1 cup, 206 g

Cassava With Creole Sauce, Puerto Rican Style ☛ Vitamin K = 9 mcg; DV = 7.5%; Serving size: 1 serving (2 pieces with sauce), 230 g

Cassava, Cooked Without Fat ☛ Vitamin K = 0.4 mcg; DV = 0.3%; Serving size: 1 piece, 20 g

Cauliflower ☛ Vitamin K = 16.6 mcg; DV = 13.8%; Serving size: 1 cup chopped, 107 g

Cauliflower Canned, Cooked Without Fat ☛ Vitamin K = 21.2 mcg; DV = 17.7%; Serving size: 1 cup, 180 g

Cauliflower Fresh or Frozen, Cooked Without Fat ☛ Vitamin K = 3 mcg; DV = 2.5%; Serving size: 1 piece, 22 g

Cauliflower, Cooked Boiled, Drained ☛ Vitamin K = 21.4 mcg; DV = 17.8%; Serving size: 1 cup , 180 g

Celeriac ☛ Vitamin K = 64 mcg; DV = 53.3%; Serving size: 1 cup, 156 g

Celeriac, Cooked ☛ Vitamin K = 66.5 mcg; DV = 55.4%; Serving size: 1 cup, pieces, 155 g

Celery ☛ Vitamin K = 29.6 mcg; DV = 24.7%; Serving size: 1 cup chopped, 101 g

Celery, Cooked Boiled, Drained ☛ Vitamin K = 56.7 mcg; DV = 47.3%; Serving size: 1 cup, diced, 150 g

Celery, Cooked Without Fat ☛ Vitamin K = 56.4 mcg; DV = 47%; Serving size: 1 cup, diced, 150 g

Celery, Creamed ☛ Vitamin K = 47.9 mcg; DV = 39.9%; Serving size: 1 cup, 228 g

Chamnamul, Cooked With Fat ☛ Vitamin K = 583.2 mcg; DV = 486%; Serving size: 1 cup, 151 g

Chamnamul, Cooked Without Fat ☛ Vitamin K = 591.2 mcg; DV = 492.7%; Serving size: 1 cup, 146 g

Channa Saag ☛ Vitamin K = 776.9 mcg; DV = 647.4%; Serving size: 1 cup, 245 g

Chard Swiss, Cooked Boiled, Drained ☛ Vitamin K = 572.8 mcg; DV = 477.3%; Serving size: 1 cup, chopped, 175 g

Chard, Cooked Without Fat ☛ Vitamin K = 471.8 mcg; DV = 393.2%; Serving size: 1 cup, stalk and leaves, 145 g

Chayote Fruit, Raw ☛ Vitamin K = 5.4 mcg; DV = 4.5%; Serving size: 1 cup, 132 g

Chicory Greens ☛ Vitamin K = 86.3 mcg; DV = 71.9%; Serving size: 1 cup, chopped, 29 g

Chinese Broccoli, Fresh or Frozen, Cooked Without Fat ☛ Vitamin K = 73.7 mcg; DV = 61.4%; Serving size: 1 cup, 88 g

Chinese Cabbage Salad With Dressing ☛ Vitamin K = 23.1 mcg; DV = 19.3%; Serving size: 1 cup, 76 g

Chinese Cabbage, Cooked Without Fat ☛ Vitamin K = 57.5 mcg; DV = 47.9%; Serving size: 1 cup, 170 g

Chinese Cabbage, Raw ☛ Vitamin K = 32.6 mcg; DV = 27.2%; Serving size: 1 cup, shredded, 76 g

Chives ☛ Vitamin K = 6.4 mcg; DV = 5.3%; Serving size: 1 tbsp chopped, 3 g

Christophine, Cooked With Fat ☛ Vitamin K = 9.6 mcg; DV = 8%; Serving size: 1 cup, 165 g

Christophine, Cooked Without Fat ☛ Vitamin K = 7.5 mcg; DV = 6.3%; Serving size: 1 cup, 160 g

Chrysanthemum ☛ Vitamin K = 87.5 mcg; DV = 72.9%; Serving size: 1 cup, 25 g

Chrysanthemum Garland, Cooked Boiled, Drained ☛ Vitamin K = 142.7 mcg; DV = 118.9%; Serving size: 1 cup, 100 g

Cilantro ☛ Vitamin K = 12.4 mcg; DV = 10.3%; Serving size: 1/4 cup, 4 g

Cobb Salad, Without Dressing ☛ Vitamin K = 35.4 mcg; DV = 29.5%; Serving size: 1 cup, 105 g

Collards ☛ Vitamin K = 157.4 mcg; DV = 131.2%; Serving size: 1 cup, chopped, 36 g

Collards, Canned, Cooked Without Fat ☛ Vitamin K = 650.4 mcg; DV = 542%; Serving size: 1 cup, canned, 162 g

Collards, Fresh or Frozen, Cooked Without Fat ☛ Vitamin K = 517.8 mcg; DV = 431.5%; Serving size: 1 cup, fresh, 128 g

Collards, Cooked Boiled, Drained ☛ Vitamin K = 772.5 mcg; DV = 643.8%; Serving size: 1 cup, chopped, 190 g

Corn Dried, Cooked ☛ Vitamin K = 2 mcg; DV = 1.7%; Serving size: 1 oz, 28 g

Corn Fritter ☛ Vitamin K = 11.8 mcg; DV = 9.8%; Serving size: 1 cup, 107 g

Corn Scalloped Or Pudding ☛ Vitamin K = 6.8 mcg; DV = 5.7%; Serving size: 1 cup, 214 g

Corn Yellow And White, Canned, Cooked Without Fat ☛ Vitamin K = 0 mcg; DV = 0%; Serving size: 1 cup, 164 g

Corn, Fresh or Frozen, Cooked With Cream Sauce ☛ Vitamin K = 1.5 mcg; DV = 1.3%; Serving size: 1 cup, 256 g

Cress Fresh, Frozen Or Canned, Cooked Without Fat ☛ Vitamin K = 513.8 mcg; DV = 428.2%; Serving size: 1 cup, 135 g

Cucumber, Peeled or Unpeeled, Raw ☛ Vitamin K = 10.2 mcg; DV = 8.5%; Serving size: 1 cup, pared, chopped, 142 g

Dandelion Greens, Cooked Boiled, Drained ☛ Vitamin K = 376.8 mcg; DV = 314%; Serving size: 1 cup, chopped, 105 g

Dandelion Greens, Cooked Without Fat ☛ Vitamin K = 573.5 mcg; DV = 477.9%; Serving size: 1 cup, chopped, 105 g

Dandelion Greens, Raw ☛ Vitamin K = 428.1 mcg; DV = 356.8%; Serving size: 1 cup, chopped, 55 g

Dasheen Boiled ☛ Vitamin K = 1.7 mcg; DV = 1.4%; Serving size: 1 cup, pieces, 142 g

Dasheen Fried ☛ Vitamin K = 7.5 mcg; DV = 6.3%; Serving size: 1 cup, pieces, 123 g

Dill Pickles ☛ Vitamin K = 6.1 mcg; DV = 5.1%; Serving size: 1 spear, small, 35 g

Drumstick Leaves, Cooked Boiled, Drained ☛ Vitamin K = 45.4 mcg; DV = 37.8%; Serving size: 1 cup, chopped, 42 g

Eggplant ☛ Vitamin K = 2.9 mcg; DV = 2.4%; Serving size: 1 cup, cubes, 82 g

Eggplant, Cooked Boiled, Drained ☛ Vitamin K = 2.9 mcg; DV = 2.4%; Serving size: 1 cup, 99 g

Eggplant, Batter-Dipped Fried ☛ Vitamin K = 18.3 mcg; DV = 15.3%; Serving size: 1 cup, 220 g

Eggplant, Cooked Without Fat ☛ Vitamin K = 6.7 mcg; DV = 5.6%; Serving size: 1 cup, 231 g

Endive ☛ Vitamin K = 115.5 mcg; DV = 96.3%; Serving size: 1 head, chopped, 50 g

Escarole, Cooked Without Fat ☛ Vitamin K = 273.4 mcg; DV = 227.8%; Serving size: 1 cup, 130 g

Escarole, Creamed ☛ Vitamin K = 220.6 mcg; DV = 183.8%; Serving size: 1 cup, 200 g

Fennel ☛ Vitamin K = 54.6 mcg; DV = 45.5%; Serving size: 1 cup, sliced, 87 g

Fennel Bulb, Cooked Without Fat ☛ Vitamin K = 209.1 mcg; DV = 174.3%; Serving size: 1 fennel bulb, 211 g

Garden Cress ☛ Vitamin K = 271 mcg; DV = 225.8%; Serving size: 1 cup, 50 g

Garlic ☛ Vitamin K = 0.1 mcg; DV = 0.1%; Serving size: 1 clove, 3 g

Ginger ☛ Vitamin K = 0 mcg; DV = 0%; Serving size: 1 tsp, 2 g

Gourd Dishcloth, Cooked Boiled, Drained ☛ Vitamin K = 3 mcg; DV = 2.5%; Serving size: 1 cup, 178 g

Gourd Dishcloth, Raw ☛ Vitamin K = 0.7 mcg; DV = 0.6%; Serving size: 1 cup, 95 g

Grape Leaves, Raw ☛ Vitamin K = 15.2 mcg; DV = 12.7%; Serving size: 1 cup, 14 g

Greek Salad, No Dressing ☛ Vitamin K = 67.7 mcg; DV = 56.4%; Serving size: 1 cup, 105 g

Green Banana Fried ☛ Vitamin K = 1.8 mcg; DV = 1.5%; Serving size: 1 slice, 23 g

Green Banana, Cooked Boiled ☛ Vitamin K = 0.3 mcg; DV = 0.3%; Serving size: 1 small, 54 g

Green Bell Peppers ☛ Vitamin K = 11 mcg; DV = 9.2%; Serving size: 1 cup, chopped, 149 g

Green Cabbage, Cooked Without Fat ☛ Vitamin K = 162 mcg; DV = 135%; Serving size: 1 cup, 150 g

Green Cauliflower ☛ Vitamin K = 12.9 mcg; DV = 10.8%; Serving size: 1 cup, 64 g

Green Leaf Lettuce ☛ Vitamin K = 45.5 mcg; DV = 37.9%; Serving size: 1 cup shredded, 36 g

Green Plantains Boiled ☛ Vitamin K = 0.2 mcg; DV = 0.2%; Serving size: 1 slice, 27 g

Green Snap Beans, Raw ☛ Vitamin K = 43 mcg; DV = 35.8%; Serving size: 1 cup, 100 g

Green Tomatoes ☛ Vitamin K = 18.2 mcg; DV = 15.2%; Serving size: 1 cup, 180 g

Greens, Canned, Cooked Without Fat ☛ Vitamin K = 860.5 mcg; DV = 717.1%; Serving size: 1 cup, 170 g

Greens, Fresh or Frozen, Cooked Without Fat ☛ Vitamin K = 739.1 mcg; DV = 615.9%; Serving size: 1 cup, 146 g

Hot Green Chili Peppers ☛ Vitamin K = 6.4 mcg; DV = 5.3%; Serving size: 1 pepper, 45 g

Hubbard Squash ☛ Vitamin K = 1.5 mcg; DV = 1.3%; Serving size: 1 cup, cubes, 116 g

Hungarian Peppers ☛ Vitamin K = 2.7 mcg; DV = 2.3%; Serving size: 1 pepper, 27 g

Iceberg Lettuce ☛ Vitamin K = 17.4 mcg; DV = 14.5%; Serving size: 1 cup shredded, 72 g

Irishmoss Seaweed ☛ Vitamin K = 0.5 mcg; DV = 0.4%; Serving size: 2 tbsp (1/8 cup), 10 g

Jalapeno Peppers ☛ Vitamin K = 16.7 mcg; DV = 13.9%; Serving size: 1 cup, sliced, 90 g

Japanese Cabbage, Style Fresh Pickled ☛ Vitamin K = 188.9 mcg; DV = 157.4%; Serving size: 1 cup, 150 g

Jute Potherb, Cooked Boiled ☛ Vitamin K = 94 mcg; DV = 78.3%; Serving size: 1 cup, 87 g

Kale ☛ Vitamin K = 506.5 mcg; DV = 422.1%; Serving size: 1 cup, chopped, 130 g

Kale, Canned, Cooked Without Fat ☛ Vitamin K = 1321.6 mcg; DV = 1101.3%; Serving size: 1 cup, canned, 163 g

Kale, Fresh or Frozen, Cooked Without Fat ☛ Vitamin K = 1054 mcg; DV = 878.3%; Serving size: 1 cup, fresh, 130 g

Kale, Cooked Boiled, Drained ☛ Vitamin K = 544.1 mcg; DV = 453.4%; Serving size: 1 cup, chopped, 130 g

Kelp Seaweed ☛ Vitamin K = 6.6 mcg; DV = 5.5%; Serving size: 2 tbsp (1/8 cup), 10 g

Ketchup ☛ Vitamin K = 0.5 mcg; DV = 0.4%; Serving size: 1 tbsp, 17 g

Kimchi ☛ Vitamin K = 65.4 mcg; DV = 54.5%; Serving size: 1 cup, 150 g

Kohlrabi ☛ Vitamin K = 0.1 mcg; DV = 0.1%; Serving size: 1 cup, 135 g

Lambsquarter, Cooked Without Fat ☛ Vitamin K = 884.7 mcg; DV = 737.3%; Serving size: 1 cup, 180 g

Lambsquarters, Cooked Boiled, Drained ☛ Vitamin K = 889.6 mcg; DV = 741.3%; Serving size: 1 cup, chopped, 180 g

Leeks ☛ Vitamin K = 41.8 mcg; DV = 34.8%; Serving size: 1 cup, 89 g

Leeks, Cooked Boiled, Drained ☛ Vitamin K = 31.5 mcg; DV = 26.3%; Serving size: 1 leek, 124 g

Lettuce Raw ☛ Vitamin K = 30 mcg; DV = 25%; Serving size: 1 cup, 125 g

Lettuce, Cooked With Fat ☛ Vitamin K = 31.6 mcg; DV = 26.3%; Serving size: 1 cup, 86 g

Lettuce, Cooked Without Fat ☛ Vitamin K = 19.4 mcg; DV = 16.2%; Serving size: 1 cup, 81 g

Lima Beans, Immature Seeds, Raw ☛ Vitamin K = 8.7 mcg; DV = 7.3%; Serving size: 1 cup, 156 g

Lotus Root, Cooked With Fat ☛ Vitamin K = 10.4 mcg; DV = 8.7%; Serving size: 1 cup, 125 g

Lotus Root, Cooked Without Fat ☛ Vitamin K = 0.1 mcg; DV = 0.1%; Serving size: 1 cup, 120 g

Luffa, Cooked With Fat ☛ Vitamin K = 76.7 mcg; DV = 63.9%; Serving size: 1 cup, 183 g

Luffa, Cooked Without Fat ☛ Vitamin K = 70.8 mcg; DV = 59%; Serving size: 1 cup, 178 g

Mushroom Asian, Cooked From Dried ☛ Vitamin K = 0 mcg; DV = 0%; Serving size: 1 cup, 145 g

Mushrooms Batter-Dipped Fried ☛ Vitamin K = 3.2 mcg; DV = 2.7%; Serving size: 1 cup, 145 g

Mushrooms, Canned, Cooked Without Fat ☛ Vitamin K = 0 mcg; DV = 0%; Serving size: 1 piece, 4 g

Mushrooms, Fresh or Frozen, Cooked Without Fat ☛ Vitamin K = 0 mcg; DV = 0%; Serving size: 1 piece, 4 g

Mushrooms Portobellos Grilled ☛ Vitamin K = 0 mcg; DV = 0%; Serving size: 1 cup sliced, 121 g

Mushrooms Shiitake, Stir-Fried ☛ Vitamin K = 0 mcg; DV = 0%; Serving size: 1 cup whole, 89 g

Mushrooms Stuffed ☛ Vitamin K = 3.3 mcg; DV = 2.8%; Serving size: 1 stuffed cap, 24 g

Mustard Cabbage, Cooked With Fat ☛ Vitamin K = 59.7 mcg; DV = 49.8%; Serving size: 1 cup, 175 g

Mustard Cabbage, Cooked Without Fat ☛ Vitamin K = 57.5 mcg; DV = 47.9%; Serving size: 1 cup, 170 g

Mustard Greens ☛ Vitamin K = 144.2 mcg; DV = 120.2%; Serving size: 1 cup, chopped, 56 g

Mustard Greens, Canned, Cooked Without Fat ☛ Vitamin K = 900.4 mcg; DV = 750.3%; Serving size: 1 cup, canned, 153 g

Mustard Greens, Fresh or Frozen, Cooked Without Fat ☛ Vitamin K = 823.9 mcg; DV = 686.6%; Serving size: 1 cup, 140 g

Mustard Greens, Cooked Boiled, Drained ☛ Vitamin K = 829.8 mcg; DV = 691.5%; Serving size: 1 cup, chopped, 140 g

New Zealand Spinach ☛ Vitamin K = 188.7 mcg; DV = 157.3%; Serving size: 1 cup, chopped, 56 g

New Zealand Spinach, Cooked Boiled, Drained ☛ Vitamin K = 525.6 mcg; DV = 438%; Serving size: 1 cup, chopped, 180 g

Nopales ☛ Vitamin K = 4.6 mcg; DV = 3.8%; Serving size: 1 cup, sliced, 86 g

Okra ☛ Vitamin K = 31.3 mcg; DV = 26.1%; Serving size: 1 cup, 100 g

Okra, Canned, Cooked Without Fat ☛ Vitamin K = 66.5 mcg; DV = 55.4%; Serving size: 1 cup, 167 g

Okra, Fresh, Frozen Or Canned, Cooked Without Fat ☛ Vitamin K = 63.7 mcg; DV = 53.1%; Serving size: 1 cup, 160 g

Okra, Cooked Boiled, Drained ☛ Vitamin K = 32 mcg; DV = 26.7%; Serving size: 1/2 cup slices, 80 g

Okra, Batter-Dipped Fried ☛ Vitamin K = 19.7 mcg; DV = 16.4%; Serving size: 1 cup, 92 g

Onion Rings, Fresh or Frozen Batter-Dipped Baked Or Fried ☛ Vitamin K = 10.4 mcg; DV = 8.7%; Serving size: 10 small rings, 48 g

Onions ☛ Vitamin K = 0.6 mcg; DV = 0.5%; Serving size: 1 cup, chopped, 160 g

Onions, Fresh or Frozen, Cooked Without Fat ☛ Vitamin K = 1.1 mcg; DV = 0.9%; Serving size: 1 cup, 210 g

Onions Dehydrated Flakes ☛ Vitamin K = 0.2 mcg; DV = 0.2%;

Serving size: 1 tbsp, 5 g

Onions Green, Fresh or Frozen, Cooked Without Fat ☞ Vitamin K = 472.4 mcg; DV = 393.7%; Serving size: 1 cup, chopped, 219 g

Onions Green, Fresh or Frozen, Cooked With Fat ☞ Vitamin K = 477.6 mcg; DV = 398%; Serving size: 1 cup, chopped, 224 g

Onions Pearl, Fresh or Frozen, Cooked ☞ Vitamin K = 0.9 mcg; DV = 0.8%; Serving size: 1 cup, 185 g

Onions Young Green Only Tops ☞ Vitamin K = 9.4 mcg; DV = 7.8%; Serving size: 1 tbsp, 6 g

Onions, Cooked Boiled, Drained ☞ Vitamin K = 1.1 mcg; DV = 0.9%; Serving size: 1 cup, 210 g

Onions, Fresh or Frozen, Creamed ☞ Vitamin K = 1.4 mcg; DV = 1.2%; Serving size: 1 cup, 228 g

Oriental Radishes ☞ Vitamin K = 0.3 mcg; DV = 0.3%; Serving size: 1 cup slices, 116 g

Palak Paneer ☞ Vitamin K = 356.2 mcg; DV = 296.8%; Serving size: 1 cup, 200 g

Palm Hearts ☞ Vitamin K = 0 mcg; DV = 0%; Serving size: 1 cup, 146 g

Parsley ☞ Vitamin K = 984 mcg; DV = 820%; Serving size: 1 cup chopped, 60 g

Parsnips, Cooked Boiled, Drained ☞ Vitamin K = 1.6 mcg; DV = 1.3%; Serving size: 1 cup slices, 156 g

Parsnips, Cooked Without Fat ☞ Vitamin K = 1.6 mcg; DV = 1.3%; Serving size: 1 cup, pieces, 156 g

Parsnips, Creamed ☞ Vitamin K = 2.3 mcg; DV = 1.9%; Serving size: 1 cup, 228 g

Pea Salad ☞ Vitamin K = 115.6 mcg; DV = 96.3%; Serving size: 1 cup,

214 g

Peas ☛ Vitamin K = 36 mcg; DV = 30%; Serving size: 1 cup, 145 g

Pepper Sweet Red, Raw ☛ Vitamin K = 0.5 mcg; DV = 0.4%; Serving size: 1 piece, 10 g

Peppers Green, Cooked Without Fat ☛ Vitamin K = 13.2 mcg; DV = 11%; Serving size: 1 cup, 136 g

Peppers Red, Cooked Without Fat ☛ Vitamin K = 6.9 mcg; DV = 5.8%; Serving size: 1 cup, 136 g

Peppers Sweet Red Freeze-Dried ☛ Vitamin K = 0.5 mcg; DV = 0.4%; Serving size: 1 tbsp, 0.4 g

Plantain Ripe Rolled In Flour Fried ☛ Vitamin K = 6.4 mcg; DV = 5.3%; Serving size: 1 piece (2-1/2" long), 45 g

Poke Greens, Cooked Without Fat ☛ Vitamin K = 166.3 mcg; DV = 138.6%; Serving size: 1 cup, 155 g

Pokeberry Shoots (Poke), Cooked Boiled, Drained ☛ Vitamin K = 178.2 mcg; DV = 148.5%; Serving size: 1 cup, 165 g

Portobellos Mushrooms ☛ Vitamin K = 0 mcg; DV = 0%; Serving size: 1 cup diced, 86 g

Potato Baked, Boiled Or Roasted ☛ Vitamin K = 4.6 mcg; DV = 3.8%; Serving size: 1 small, 230 g

Potato Flour ☛ Vitamin K = 0 mcg; DV = 0%; Serving size: 1 cup, 160 g

Potatoes French Fried ☛ Vitamin K = 2.9 mcg; DV = 2.4%; Serving size: 20 strip, 130 g

Potatoes Hash Brown Pan-Fried In Canola Oil ☛ Vitamin K = 25.5 mcg; DV = 21.3%; Serving size: 1 cup prepared, 130 g

Potatoes Hash Brown Unprepared ☛ Vitamin K = 0.6 mcg; DV = 0.5%; Serving size: 1 cup unprepared, 159 g

Potatoes Mashed Dehydrated Flakes ☛ Vitamin K = 5.2 mcg; DV = 4.3%; Serving size: 1 cup, 60 g

Pumpkin, Fresh or Frozen, Cooked Without Fat ☛ Vitamin K = 2 mcg; DV = 1.7%; Serving size: 1 cup, 245 g

Pumpkin Leaves, Cooked Boiled, Drained ☛ Vitamin K = 76.7 mcg; DV = 63.9%; Serving size: 1 cup, 71 g

Pumpkin, Canned ☛ Vitamin K = 39.2 mcg; DV = 32.7%; Serving size: 1 cup, 245 g

Pumpkin, Raw ☛ Vitamin K = 1.3 mcg; DV = 1.1%; Serving size: 1 cup, 116 g

Radicchio ☛ Vitamin K = 102.1 mcg; DV = 85.1%; Serving size: 1 cup, shredded, 40 g

Radish Daikon, Cooked With Fat ☛ Vitamin K = 5.8 mcg; DV = 4.8%; Serving size: 1 cup, 153 g

Radish Daikon, Cooked Without Fat ☛ Vitamin K = 0.4 mcg; DV = 0.3%; Serving size: 1 cup, 147 g

Radishes ☛ Vitamin K = 1.5 mcg; DV = 1.3%; Serving size: 1 cup slices, 116 g

Radishes Oriental Dried ☛ Vitamin K = 5.2 mcg; DV = 4.3%; Serving size: 1 cup, 116 g

Red Cabbage ☛ Vitamin K = 34 mcg; DV = 28.3%; Serving size: 1 cup, chopped, 89 g

Red Cabbage, Cooked Without Fat ☛ Vitamin K = 71 mcg; DV = 59.2%; Serving size: 1 cup, 150 g

Red Chili Peppers ☛ Vitamin K = 6.3 mcg; DV = 5.3%; Serving size: 1 pepper, 45 g

Red Leaf Lettuce ☛ Vitamin K = 39.3 mcg; DV = 32.8%; Serving size: 1 cup shredded, 28 g

Romaine Lettuce ☛ Vitamin K = 48.2 mcg; DV = 40.2%; Serving size: 1 cup shredded, 47 g

Rutabaga, Cooked Without Fat ☛ Vitamin K = 0.3 mcg; DV = 0.3%; Serving size: 1 cup, pieces, 170 g

Salsify, Cooked Boiled, Drained ☛ Vitamin K = 0.4 mcg; DV = 0.3%; Serving size: 1 cup, sliced, 135 g

Salsify, Cooked With Fat ☛ Vitamin K = 2.5 mcg; DV = 2.1%; Serving size: 1 cup, 140 g

Salsify, Cooked Without Fat ☛ Vitamin K = 0.4 mcg; DV = 0.3%; Serving size: 1 cup, 135 g

Sambar Vegetable Stew ☛ Vitamin K = 17.9 mcg; DV = 14.9%; Serving size: 1 cup, 248 g

Sauerkraut ☛ Vitamin K = 18.5 mcg; DV = 15.4%; Serving size: 1 cup, 142 g

Savoy Cabbage ☛ Vitamin K = 48.2 mcg; DV = 40.2%; Serving size: 1 cup, shredded, 70 g

Savoy Cabbage, Cooked Without Fat ☛ Vitamin K = 103.2 mcg; DV = 86%; Serving size: 1 cup, 145 g

Scallop Squash ☛ Vitamin K = 4.3 mcg; DV = 3.6%; Serving size: 1 cup slices, 130 g

Seaweed Agar, Raw ☛ Vitamin K = 0.2 mcg; DV = 0.2%; Serving size: 2 tbsp (1/8 cup), 10 g

Seaweed, Raw ☛ Vitamin K = 15.4 mcg; DV = 12.8%; Serving size: 1 cup, 80 g

Serrano Peppers ☛ Vitamin K = 12.4 mcg; DV = 10.3%; Serving size: 1 cup, chopped, 105 g

Shallots ☛ Vitamin K = 0.1 mcg; DV = 0.1%; Serving size: 1 tbsp chopped, 10 g

Shallots Freeze-Dried ☞ Vitamin K = 0 mcg; DV = 0%; Serving size: 1 tbsp, 0.9 g

Sour Pickled Cucumber ☞ Vitamin K = 72.9 mcg; DV = 60.8%; Serving size: 1 cup, 155 g

Spaghetti Squash ☞ Vitamin K = 0.9 mcg; DV = 0.8%; Serving size: 1 cup, cubes, 101 g

Spinach ☞ Vitamin K = 144.9 mcg; DV = 120.8%; Serving size: 1 cup, 30 g

Spinach, Canned, Cooked Without Fat ☞ Vitamin K = 985.9 mcg; DV = 821.6%; Serving size: 1 cup, canned, 214 g

Spinach, Fresh or Frozen, Cooked Without Fat ☞ Vitamin K = 883.6 mcg; DV = 736.3%; Serving size: 1 cup, fresh, 180 g

Spinach Salad, No Dressing ☞ Vitamin K = 257.4 mcg; DV = 214.5%; Serving size: 1 cup, 74 g

Spinach Souffle ☞ Vitamin K = 172 mcg; DV = 143.3%; Serving size: 1 cup, 136 g

Spinach, Cooked Boiled, Drained ☞ Vitamin K = 468.9 mcg; DV = 390.8%; Serving size: 1/2 cup, 95 g

Spinach, Canned, Creamed ☞ Vitamin K = 583.4 mcg; DV = 486.2%; Serving size: 1 cup, 200 g

Spinach, Fresh or Frozen, Creamed ☞ Vitamin K = 582.6 mcg; DV = 485.5%; Serving size: 1 cup, 200 g

Spring Onions ☞ Vitamin K = 207 mcg; DV = 172.5%; Serving size: 1 cup, chopped, 100 g

Squash Fritter Or Cake ☞ Vitamin K = 3.1 mcg; DV = 2.6%; Serving size: 1 fritter, 24 g

Squash Spaghetti, Cooked Without Fat ☞ Vitamin K = 1.2 mcg; DV = 1%; Serving size: 1 cup, cooked, 155 g

Squash Summer, Canned, Creamed ☛ Vitamin K = 4.6 mcg; DV = 3.8%; Serving size: 1 cup, 217 g

Squash Summer, Fresh or Frozen, Creamed ☛ Vitamin K = 5.2 mcg; DV = 4.3%; Serving size: 1 cup, 217 g

Squash Winter All Varieties, Cooked ☛ Vitamin K = 9 mcg; DV = 7.5%; Serving size: 1 cup, cubes, 205 g

Sun-Dried Hot Chile Peppers ☛ Vitamin K = 40 mcg; DV = 33.3%; Serving size: 1 cup, 37 g

Sun-Dried Tomatoes ☛ Vitamin K = 23.2 mcg; DV = 19.3%; Serving size: 1 cup, 54 g

Sweet Onions ☛ Vitamin K = 0.4 mcg; DV = 0.3%; Serving size: 1 nlea serving, 148 g

Sweet Pickled Cucumbers ☛ Vitamin K = 37.7 mcg; DV = 31.4%; Serving size: 1/2 cup, chopped, 80 g

Sweet Pickled Relish ☛ Vitamin K = 12.6 mcg; DV = 10.5%; Serving size: 1 tbsp, 15 g

Sweet Potato Candied ☛ Vitamin K = 2 mcg; DV = 1.7%; Serving size: 1 piece, 45 g

Sweet Potato Casserole Or Mashed ☛ Vitamin K = 4.8 mcg; DV = 4%; Serving size: 1 cup, 250 g

Sweet Potato Cooked Without Fat ☛ Vitamin K = 1.8 mcg; DV = 1.5%; Serving size: 1 small, 80 g

Sweet Potato Fries, Fried, From Fresh or Frozen Fried ☛ Vitamin K = 8.7 mcg; DV = 7.3%; Serving size: 1 fry, any cut, 50 g

Sweet Potato Fries, Baked, From Fresh or Frozen ☛ Vitamin K = 6.4 mcg; DV = 5.3%; Serving size: 1 fry, any cut, 50 g

Sweet Potato Leaves, Raw ☛ Vitamin K = 105.8 mcg; DV = 88.2%; Serving size: 1 cup, chopped, 35 g

Sweet Potato, Cooked Candied, Home-Made ☛ Vitamin K = 2.2 mcg; DV = 1.8%; Serving size: 1 piece, 105 g

Sweet Potatoes ☛ Vitamin K = 2.4 mcg; DV = 2%; Serving size: 1 cup, cubes, 133 g

Sweet Red Bell Peppers ☛ Vitamin K = 7.3 mcg; DV = 6.1%; Serving size: 1 cup, chopped, 149 g

Swiss Chard ☛ Vitamin K = 298.8 mcg; DV = 249%; Serving size: 1 cup, 36 g

Tannier, Cooked ☛ Vitamin K = 2.7 mcg; DV = 2.3%; Serving size: 1 cup, 190 g

Taro Leaves, Raw ☛ Vitamin K = 30.4 mcg; DV = 25.3%; Serving size: 1 cup, 28 g

Taro raw ☛ Vitamin K = 1 mcg; DV = 0.8%; Serving size: 1 cup, sliced, 104 g

Thistle Leaves, Cooked With Fat ☛ Vitamin K = 683.2 mcg; DV = 569.3%; Serving size: 1 cup, 185 g

Thistle Leaves, Cooked Without Fat ☛ Vitamin K = 685.1 mcg; DV = 570.9%; Serving size: 1 cup, 180 g

Tomatillos ☛ Vitamin K = 10.3 mcg; DV = 8.6%; Serving size: 3 medium, 102 g

Tomatoes ☛ Vitamin K = 11.8 mcg; DV = 9.8%; Serving size: 1 cup cherry tomatoes, 149 g

Tomatoes Crushed, Canned ☛ Vitamin K = 6.4 mcg; DV = 5.3%; Serving size: 1/2 cup, 121 g

Tomatoes Green, Fresh or Frozen, Cooked ☛ Vitamin K = 17.8 mcg; DV = 14.8%; Serving size: 1 small, 75 g

Tomatoes Red Ripe, Canned In Tomato Juice ☛ Vitamin K = 6.2 mcg; DV = 5.2%; Serving size: 1 cup, 240 g

Tomatoes Red, Fresh or Frozen Fried ☛ Vitamin K = 15 mcg; DV = 12.5%; Serving size: 1 small, 75 g

Tomatoes, Fresh or Frozen Broiled ☛ Vitamin K = 1.4 mcg; DV = 1.2%; Serving size: 1 cherry, 14 g

Tomatoes, Fresh or Frozen Scalloped ☛ Vitamin K = 21.9 mcg; DV = 18.3%; Serving size: 1 cup, 235 g

Tomatoes, Fresh or Frozen Stewed ☛ Vitamin K = 7.1 mcg; DV = 5.9%; Serving size: 1 tomato, 114 g

Turnip, Canned, Cooked Without Fat ☛ Vitamin K = 0.2 mcg; DV = 0.2%; Serving size: 1 cup, pieces, 155 g

Turnip, Fresh or Frozen, Cooked Without Fat ☛ Vitamin K = 0.2 mcg; DV = 0.2%; Serving size: 1 cup, pieces, 155 g

Turnip Greens ☛ Vitamin K = 138.1 mcg; DV = 115.1%; Serving size: 1 cup, chopped, 55 g

Turnip Greens, From Canned, Cooked Without Fat ☛ Vitamin K = 453.2 mcg; DV = 377.7%; Serving size: 1 cup, canned, 159 g

Turnip Greens, Fresh or Frozen, Cooked Without Fat ☛ Vitamin K = 525.7 mcg; DV = 438.1%; Serving size: 1 cup, fresh, 144 g

Turnip Greens With Roots, Canned, Cooked Without Fat ☛ Vitamin K = 223.1 mcg; DV = 185.9%; Serving size: 1 cup, 163 g

Turnip Greens With Roots, Fresh or Frozen, Cooked Without Fat ☛ Vitamin K = 285.7 mcg; DV = 238.1%; Serving size: 1 cup, 163 g

Turnip Greens With Roots, Canned, Cooked With Fat ☛ Vitamin K = 225.3 mcg; DV = 187.8%; Serving size: 1 cup, 168 g

Turnip Greens With Roots, Fresh or Frozen, Cooked With Fat ☛ Vitamin K = 288 mcg; DV = 240%; Serving size: 1 cup, 168 g

Turnip Greens, Cooked Boiled, Drained ☛ Vitamin K = 529.3 mcg; DV = 441.1%; Serving size: 1 cup, chopped, 144 g

Turnips ☛ Vitamin K = 0.1 mcg; DV = 0.1%; Serving size: 1 cup, cubes, 130 g

Turnips, Cooked Boiled, Drained ☛ Vitamin K = 0.2 mcg; DV = 0.2%; Serving size: 1 cup, cubes, 156 g

Wakame ☛ Vitamin K = 0.5 mcg; DV = 0.4%; Serving size: 2 tbsp (1/8 cup), 10 g

Water Chestnut ☛ Vitamin K = 0.5 mcg; DV = 0.4%; Serving size: 1 cup, 158 g

Watercress ☛ Vitamin K = 85 mcg; DV = 70.8%; Serving size: 1 cup, chopped, 34 g

Watercress, Cooked With Fat ☛ Vitamin K = 334.3 mcg; DV = 278.6%; Serving size: 1 cup, 142 g

Watercress, Cooked Without Fat ☛ Vitamin K = 340.4 mcg; DV = 283.7%; Serving size: 1 cup, 137 g

Waxgourd, Cooked Boiled, Drained ☛ Vitamin K = 4.9 mcg; DV = 4.1%; Serving size: 1 cup, cubes, 175 g

Yam ☛ Vitamin K = 3.5 mcg; DV = 2.9%; Serving size: 1 cup, cubes, 150 g

Yam, Cooked Puerto Rican ☛ Vitamin K = 3.2 mcg; DV = 2.7%; Serving size: 1 cup, 140 g

Yambean (Jicama), Raw ☛ Vitamin K = 0.4 mcg; DV = 0.3%; Serving size: 1 cup slices, 120 g

Yellow Onions ☛ Vitamin K = 18.8 mcg; DV = 15.7%; Serving size: 1 cup chopped, 87 g

Yuca Fries ☛ Vitamin K = 25.1 mcg; DV = 20.9%; Serving size: 1 cup, 140 g

Zucchini ☛ Vitamin K = 5.3 mcg; DV = 4.4%; Serving size: 1 cup, chopped, 124 g

HEALTH AND NUTRITION WEBSITES

A PATIENT'S GUIDE TO TAKING WARFARIN:

www.heart.org/en/health-topics/arrhythmia/prevention--treat-ment-of-arrhythmia/a-patients-guide-to-taking-warfarin

GUIDE TO WARFARIN USE:

www.ihtc.org/userfiles/file/resources/Patient%20Manual%20-%20Warfarin.pdf

BLOOD THINNER PILLS: YOUR GUIDE TO USING THEM SAFELY

www.ahrq.gov/patients-consumers/diagnosis-treatment/treat-ments/btpills/btpills.html

CENTERS FOR DISEASE CONTROL AND PREVENTION:

https://www.cdc.gov/stroke/index.htm

Made in the USA
Las Vegas, NV
13 January 2024

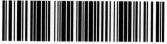

84327775R00109